Simone Algeri
Claus D. Stobäus

Workshops for aggressors: Interfaces between Social Education, Health and Nursing

Simone Algeri
Claus D. Stobäus

Workshops for aggressors: Interfaces between Social Education, Health and Nursing

Repercussions of workshops for educating abusive guardians: Interfaces between social education, health and nursing

ScienciaScripts

Imprint

Cover image: www.ingimage.com

This book is a translation from the original published under ISBN 978-3-330-77287-8.

Publisher:
Sciencia Scripts
is a trademark of
Dodo Books Indian Ocean Ltd. and OmniScriptum S.R.L publishing group

120 High Road, East Finchley, London, N2 9ED, United Kingdom
Str. Armeneasca 28/1, office 1, Chisinau MD-2012, Republic of Moldova, Europe
Managing Directors: Ieva Konstantinova, Victoria Ursu
info@omniscriptum.com

Printed at: see last page
ISBN: 978-620-8-64576-2

INDICE

SIMONEALGERI

Nurse, Associate Professor at the Maternal and Child Department of the School of Nursing/UFRGS. Specialist in Mental Health and Psychiatry at the Federal University of Rio Grande do Sul (UFRGS). Master's in Nursing from UFRGS. PhD in Education from PUC/RS. Effective member of the Child Protection Program at the Hospital de Clinicas de Porto Alegre. Coordinator of the Extension Project Care and Prevention for Children Victims of Violence.

CLAUS DIETER STOBAUS

Doctor, Full Professor at the Pontifical Catholic University of Rio Grande do Sul. Master in Education from the Federal University of Rio Grande do Sul (UFRGS). PhD in Human Sciences - Education from UFRGS. Post-Doctorate in Psychology from the Universidad Autonoma de Madrid - Spain Senior Educator of the ATLS - Advanced Trauma Life Support Program, for Region XIV (2010-2016), and Educator of the ATCN - Advanced Trauma Course for Nurses.

To my daughter ROBERTA and my nephews GIORDANO, VICENZO, MARCELLO AND ANTONELLA who are the hope of a new era, showing that life has more possibilities than limits.

1 INTRODUCTION

The research I carried out as a Doctoral Thesis in Education consisted of an approach to violence, more specifically through the testimonies of aggressor mothers, responsible for children, within the area of Health Education.

I believe that studying the phenomenon of violence by associating it with Education and Health makes it possible to face it as a challenge for the 21st century, since I have always considered it to be a serious collective health problem.

For me, the subject of violence is now very present in everyday life, especially in the media, but also in the daily work of those who care for children and adolescents, and needs to be studied more.

Therefore, this area of knowledge is the subject of multiple investigations, as it generates countless controversies and polemics; however, there is an undeniable current reality: the increase in the different forms of violence present in contemporary societies.

In my work with interdisciplinary teams for more than ten years, I have tried to delve deeper into the issue of intra-family violence, and this has been important since the consequences profoundly affect the health and quality of life of the people involved. In this way, I have seen a growing demand for children subjected to various forms of violence by their caregivers, treated in public health services and often unnoticed by professionals, showing that they are unprepared for the frequency and magnitude of this phenomenon.

Intrafamily violence is independent of culture, race or creed, since it has appeared frequently in human history, demonstrating the difficulties in understanding it and trying to remove it from everyday family life. I believe that if there isn't a process of intervention from a more social and human perspective, more coherent with the individual and collective experiences of people in situations of intrafamily violence, it will be more difficult for them to cope and the consequences will be worse.

Thus, I understand that the issue of children exposed to intrafamily violence is socially relevant and so, based on my experiences, I developed this research in the form of a Doctoral Thesis, addressing the perceptions of those responsible for the children in this case, the mothers, about the reasons that lead them to physically assault their children, verifying the repercussions of the workshops of which these subjects are part.

I currently teach Nursing in Child Care at the Nursing School of the Federal University of Rio Grande do Sul, Brazil, and one of my activities consists of holding workshops once a week with families of children in situations of intrafamily violence. These workshops take place in a public hospital in Porto Alegre, which has an interdisciplinary team made up of a pediatrician, psychiatrist, psychologist, nurse, social worker, recreationalist and a representative from the Public Prosecutor's Office, as well as trainees from the fields of Medicine, Nursing, Psychology and Social Work.

I have been an active member of this institutional team since the workshops were conceived, set up and implemented.

Thus, based on the testimonies of the five aggressor mothers interviewed for this research and the analysis of the work carried out in the workshops, I sought to understand how the workshop, as an educational methodology, helps aggressor guardians to modify violent behavior towards their children.

I hope that this study will help to propose guidelines that will make educational actions possible for those responsible for the children, in relation to transforming the practice of hitting children as a form of education, which is so common in Brazil.

I believe that better preparation for nursing action with families who have children in situations of violence has become a major challenge that nurses have had to face ever since they were trained, and one that deserves more and more in-depth study, by looking at social, educational, philosophical, historical and cultural issues, among others.

I think that by looking for these subsidies in the Doctorate in Education course at the Pontifical Catholic University of Rio Grande do Sul (PUCRS), and developing this study with a qualitative approach, I have broadened my horizons, in the sense of looking for possibilities for discussion, with repercussions for my teaching and care practice, with my students, as well as with the children, adolescents and their families who make up the population I care for, with the concern of avoiding stereotypes and misinformation.

I believe that tackling the problem of violence from the social perspective of education and health requires an awareness of the individual as a social element, as well as of society as a whole.

In order for this to happen, it is necessary to provide health and education professionals with intervention tools to enable alternative ways of coping, such as workshops to reduce, eradicate and prevent intrafamily violence.

I therefore hope that by sharing our experiences and the knowledge produced in the workshops in this thesis, I can contribute to society in general and to teaching and care professionals in particular.

2. CONTEXTUALIZING VIOLENCE

Authors who are concerned with the phenomenon of violence, such as Caminha (2000), Farinatti (19931), Heller (1994) and Santos (1999), understand that its nature should be considered highly complex and highly diverse. Sharing this idea, I understand that violence is an act that causes harm to a person, and has long been a constant in the daily lives of many Brazilian families. In particular, violence against children is a phenomenon that is increasingly present in our reality. However, it is not a recent practice; it is as old as the history of humanity itself. In different historical periods and in different cultures, children have been conceived in different ways, thus giving different connotations to situations of violence against them.

As Jaeger (2003, p. 36) points out, violent punitive practices towards children are not a recent phenomenon in our society. It is the way we perceive them that has changed. Since the family, family relationships and childhood have been better understood and studied, this phenomenon has become more visible and, at times, more visible than at others. We must ask ourselves to what extent these practices constitute an action characteristic of child education or violence against children.

In line with Maldonado (1997), I see violence as the use of words or actions that harm or hurt people. The unfair and abusive use of power, as well as the use of force that results in injury, suffering, torture or death, also constitute violence.

Violence against children in the family context is not the only form of violence practiced against them, but it is one of the most frequent, as it is seen as an educational practice. There is a culture of violence understood as a form of education. This concept is strongly associated with the notion that children are the property of their parents, who believe that they have the right to life and death over their children. As Blay (2000) points out, many cases of children being abused by their guardians in public go unpunished, as it is difficult for anyone to intervene in such a case.

The results of my Master's thesis, defended at the Graduate Program of the Nursing School of the Federal University of Rio Grande do Sul (UFRGS), showed that, in the sample of 50 families surveyed, the mother was the main caregiver and, at the same time, the biggest aggressor.

Azevedo and Guerra (2001, p.13) state:

> We live in a culture where hitting children has been and continues to be recognized as a parental right, for the good of the children. Progress has already been made in banning moderate and cruel punishment, either through the 1990 Statute of the Child and Adolescent, in its article 5, or in the 1940 Penal Code (article 1361), as they are forms of abuse of parental disciplinary power.

The authors go on to point out that (p. 13):

> We live in a country where parents have a mania for hitting their children, under the false pretense that it is for their own good. Unfortunately, however, we still haven't managed to abolish what we consider to be a real national craze: that of hitting children, either with the hand (spanking, slapping...) or with the most varied instruments and objects (belts, ropes, slippers, shoes, clogs, sticks, slaps...). Since the dawn of our history, Brazilian families have in one way or another resorted to beating their children under the dubious pretext of disciplining them.

Azevedo and Guerra (2001) also point out that, when analyzing the issue of hitting children, some considerations need to be made. The first is why? On a common sense level, two answers are usually the most frequent: to discipline them, i.e. to control them, to dominate them by subjecting them to a certain order that is in line with the functioning of the family or society in general, and to punish them, i.e. to punish them for real faults or those they have supposedly committed. The result, in both cases, is the practice of hitting the child, but the intentionality of the action seems to be different, which gives it a more preventive nature when it comes to disciplining, and a more punitive nature when it comes to punishing.

According to these authors, when trying to define what it means to beat children, there is no single answer, as the means and ways used have varied over time and space. Despite the diversity that stems from the varying conceptions of what it means to raise children, there are some factors that the aforementioned authors note can be analyzed:

- all forms of hitting children are practices aimed at the child's body;
- the real or professed purpose can be either to discipline or to punish;
- all practices that affect the child's body produce physical pain;
- all practices can be distributed along a *continuum* of severity, according to the nature of the consequences in the short, medium and long term;
- although, throughout humanity, many of these practices have been applied to

slaves, Indians, servants, women, the mentally ill and the elderly, children and adolescents are still the only ones for whom the principle that they need to be beaten in order to learn to be people is defended.

Newell (1989) emphasizes that any action that causes physical pain to a child, from a simple slap to a fatal beating, represents a single *continuum of* violence. This author states that corporal punishment of children is considered violence, even the mildest punishment, insofar as all corporal punishment, in order to have this character, must imply the concept of physical pain.

Azevedo and Guerra (2001, p. 27), when discussing beating as a way of educating, state that:

> So the question we asked ourselves - "Is hitting your children a way of educating them?" will receive different answers depending on whether or not you understand hitting your children as violence. For many, it is only violence if it involves immoderate or cruel punishment, as they conservatively see the application of the Solomon proverb as educational: "Do not spare a child correction: if you punish him with a rod, he will not die" (Proverbs 23:13). For others, any punitive measure that affects the child's body can and should be considered violence, insofar as it causes physical pain. Our position, therefore, is that hitting children as domestic violence should be opposed, as it is not a way of educating them, but of diseducating them.

The Italian Help Center for Abused Children and Families in Crisis defines physical violence as physical abuse in which children or adolescents are subjected to aggression by those close to them, with physical consequences such as skin, eye and visceral injuries, fractures, burns, permanent injuries and death (Cirillo and Di Blasio 1989).

In a study by Algeri (2001), the results showed that many of the children investigated had different types of physical injuries, as well as behavioral and social alterations. Among the instruments used to hurt them, the following were found: wooden stick, leather belt, whip, sledgehammer, electric wire, slipper. As one of the mothers reported in the study (p.57*), "I think I have every right to treat my daughter the way I want"*.

Centeville, Cabral and Atadia (1997, p.102), in a study carried out on the incidence and types of punishments applied by parents or guardians to schoolchildren in the city of Campinas, concluded that, most of the time, traditional punishments are understood by parents as a form of education and are not applied with the aim of causing harm. They report that:

> For physical violence and being beaten, the instruments used were the most diverse: spanking, pinching, whipping, wooden spoon, shoe, stick, rope, baseball bat, telephone wire, punch, slap, shotgun shot to the foot, punches to the face or other parts of the body, clog, belt, slipper, ear pulling, iron wire, stick, hose, kneeling on corn, beans and bottle caps, being tied to the foot of the bed, pepper in the mouth. cold water on the face.

Authors such as Guerra (1985), Muza (1994), Biehl (1997), Santos and Algeri (1994) and Algeri (2001) report that the history of children, throughout the process of civilization, has been permeated by various forms of violence, such as slavery, abandonment, mutilation, filicide and beatings.

Gauer (1999), Balestreri (1999) and Santos (1999) state that since today's society is extremely violent, more intense and perverse forms of this phenomenon are generated. Thus, to the extent that violence is incorporated into everyday life, society is often permissive, complicit and even encourages it.

According to Santos (1996, 1999), violence is defined as a cultural and historical phenomenon. He emphasizes that the widespread expansion of violence in society, within a process known as globalization, takes on various forms and affects social groups, including the family, in its domestic context.

According to Minayo (1992, p. 263), "violence is a historical construction that has the face of the society that engenders it". Based on this statement, it is understood that it is in the asymmetrical relationships between adults and children, between husbands and wives, which are socially determined, that the foundations of the production of family violence can be found, which is perpetuated by external examples and, undoubtedly, by a great deal of ignorance. It is behaviour that occurs in the collective and private spheres, constituting structural violence, and in interpersonal relationships it is seen as natural, even historical, and that, like the order of things, it is organized in society itself.

Minayo (1994) points out that in Brazil, population-based studies show that approximately 33% of children and adolescents suffer violent acts within their families. It is therefore difficult to recognize, as it is perpetrated against the most vulnerable members of the family group, i.e. women and children, as Muza (1994), Barudy (1997), Camargo and Buralli (1998) and Morais (1999) point out.

It should be noted that the family, a group constituted as such, is the basic nucleus of a child's formation. As the primary nucleus of the individual's socialization, it is responsible for transmitting values, habits and customs.

The family, in contemporary times, is undergoing various transformations, i.e. it is a structure that has been changing according to social, cultural and historical contexts. The role of the nuclear family, based on a few individuals and the intimate coexistence of domestic space, has replaced the old extended families, based on a broad kinship network, which mixed its functionality with that of rural production and trade in goods. Today, the family is based on privacy, a restricted space for affective personal relationships, in which the number of members and their ties have been restricted.

Nowadays, there are various forms of family organization, such as single-parent families, independent productions, reconstituted families, same-sex couples, among others. So, I think that these new forms of family composition affect the dynamics of relationships, which, in my perception, can be, in a way, an indicator of difficulties. After all, these changes create a new context of power relations and inter-relationships, a different universe of expectations and subjective representations within the family.

The concept of intrafamily violence refers not only to the physical space in which the violence takes place, but also to the relationships in which it is constructed and carried out.

Intrafamily violence expresses dynamics of power and affection, in which relationships of subordination and domination are present. In these relationships between men and women, parents and children, of different generations, people are in opposite positions, often playing rigid roles and creating their own dynamic, different for each family group. I understand that intrafamily violence can manifest itself in various ways and with varying degrees of severity, and that these forms of violence do not occur in isolation, but are part of a growing sequence of episodes that affect children in particular, on a continuous basis, with significant repercussions on their health.

For Azevedo and Guerra (1998, p. 32), any act of violence against children is a denial of their right "[...] to be treated as subjects and persons in a peculiar condition of development". It should be emphasized that the subject of intrafamily violence also includes specific concepts of physical, psychological, sexual and neglect violence. Physical violence, according to Guerra (1985, p. 161), "[...] is the use of physical force against a child in a non-accidental way, causing various types of injury and being perpetrated by a father, mother, stepfather or stepmother".

Psychological violence is defined by Deslandes (1994b, p. 15) "[...] as the negative interference of an adult or older person on the child's social competence, producing a pattern of destructive behavior". Among the most common ways in which it is practiced are denial, isolation and verbal aggression.

Sexual violence is understood by Azevedo and Guerra (1989, p. 42) "[...] as any sexual act or game, hetero or homosexual relationship, between one or more adults and a child under the age of 18, the purpose of which is to sexually stimulate the child or to use the child to obtain stimulation about themselves or someone else".

Negligence is explained by Azevedo and Guerra (1989, p. 41) "as the fact that the family fails to provide for the physical and emotional needs of a child or adolescent". It is believed that behind violence in the family lies a model of education that aims to break the child's will and stifle what is alive in them in order to transform them into a docile and obedient being.

I realize that violence often occurs in a private space, in the home sweet home, a place of unrestricted power, in which adult-centric relationships are exercised authoritatively by parents who judge, through the ideal of paternal love, what is best, what "is for their own good". Thus, the use of corporal punishment, spanking and whipping are seen as normal, socially acceptable and used as justifications for correction, being disciplinary acts, always supported by the figure of paternal power, as evidenced in research carried out (ALGERI, 2001, p. 10).

I agree that, through the power relationship between parents and their children, there seems to be a clear link between subjection in the form of discipline, which often justifies the use of aggression to any degree of violence, and the use of violence as a means to an end. In other words, parents want their children to be healthy, normal and productive individuals. Thus, in our culture, which uses adult-centric power, children are hurt, beaten and even murdered by adults, whose basic function would be to protect them and defend their lives.

For psychiatrists Kaplan and Sadock (1997), child abuse is a medical-social disease that has taken on epidemic proportions and encompasses a widespread pattern of education in the population. In comments on the child protection campaign launched by Rede RBS in its newspaper Zero Hora (2003), it was pointed out that around 18,000 children are beaten every day in Brazil, with at least 100 dying every day. Of these, half are killed in their own homes. According to Corsi (1995, p. 31), "approximately 50% of families suffer or have suffered from violence between their members, which raises family violence to the status of a social problem".

3. FAMILIES OF CHILDREN SUBJECTED TO INTRAFAMILY VIOLENCE

For Nitschke (1999, p. 41), "to talk about family is to dive into waters of different and varied meanings for people, depending on where they live, their culture and also their religious and philosophical orientation, among other aspects".

In line with this author's proposal, it can be said that every human being has their own meaning of family which is intrinsically linked to their experiential reality.

We also have to consider other notions relating to family. Osòrio (1996, p. 14) says that "family is not an expression that can be conceptualized, but only described", while Morais (1999, p. 50) says that "nowadays we can't say that family is a single concept". Another author, Engels (1971, p. 67), associates the word familia with *famulus*, which means "domestic slave". The familia then referred to the group of slaves belonging to the same owner. For him, the modern family "[...] contains the groan not only of slavery, but of servitude as well".

Taking into account the opinions mentioned above, it is believed that the possible structures of family systems affect and modify the dynamics of the relationships between its members. All families go through transactional stages that make up their life cycle, in which crises arise and the family needs to reorganize itself in order to bring about change and growth (ENGELS, 1971; OS0RIO, 1996; BIEHL, 1997). It is therefore in the daily life of the family that children learn the meaning of living, develop emotional relationships and, through them, form their personalities. Each family is organized in a unique way and reacts to different situations, in other words, the family scene is shaped by socio-economic, political and cultural determinants (GUERRA, 1985; FARINATTI, 1993; SANTOSE ALGERI, 1994).

The unequal relationships between men and women, parents and children, teachers and students, as well as those between professionals in the context of work, have been highlighted throughout history in the arts, philosophy, religion and other sciences. In the sphere of the home, according to Assis (1991, p. 33), "the relationship established between family members in a violent home has links that bind all its components, not just the abusive act, but constantly feeding it".

According to Goldani (1994), the Brazilian family has undergone profound changes as a result of an extensive recession, increased concentration of income, growing poverty, the incapacity and bankruptcy of the state; this has an influence on family relationships in all population groups.

We can see that in Brazil, the family model evolved from the patriarchal family to the conjugal family. The conjugal, modern, nuclear family, made up of parents and children or at least one of the parents, has become the current hegemonic standard. It is the setting in which people reproduce and are socialized, impregnated with culture, morals and prevailing values, where gender and power relations are established and in which people get hurt, produce and reproduce violent relations.

Can this family be considered a model? I believe so, because the family is the primary reproductive nucleus of asymmetrical, violent, power-based relationships. After all, child victimization is common to the evolution and history of human civilization. It is within the family that a child is punished, a method that is socially learned and culturally passed down through generations. The family is an important factor in the biopsychosocial development of children, adults and society; violence against children is therefore a form of social relationship linked to the way in which individuals produce their existential conditions in our culture, supported by the exercise of violence itself. It is worth highlighting the thinking of Bellini (2002, p. 231), who emphasizes:

> The complexity of the family is expressed in the relationships between its members and society. It is a living world where different subjects construct their subjectivity in relationships of dispute and solidarity. Within the family, actions of discipline and subordination are developed, as well as freedom, expression and differentiation.

Meneghel (1996, p. 12), when drawing up a profile of mistreating/abused families, found that women who are mistreated by their husbands often abuse their children: "[...] in these families, the woman who is mistreated by her husband is usually the adult who mistreats her children, in a cycle where the one who has the most power hurts the who are in a lower hierarchical position, and so on and so forth".

Studies indicate that violence against children and adolescents is present in all socioeconomic categories, regardless of race, color, creed or culture. Some authors (MENEGHEL, 1996; FARINATTI, 1992; CAMINHA, 1999; SANTOS, 1998; ALGERI,

2001) who have characterized the profile of families with intrafamily violence are unanimous in describing that male aggressors can be found in different social classes, ethnic and religious groups, with a low tolerance threshold for frustration, and who mask their aggressive behavior outside the family environment. The women in these families are generally depressed, have low self-esteem and are at high risk of drug and alcohol addiction. They are submissive, passive and powerless; they are isolated from friends and the community and constantly lose the ability to protect themselves and their children.

These authors report that families with neglect, physical or psychological violence have parents who tend to hide the traumatic injuries to the child, giving unconvincing, contradictory justifications for the injuries and other problems. These are parents who show apathy and indifference towards their children, using a very harsh way of raising them; they treat the child harshly, humiliating them and downgrading their potential. They describe their children as "bad", "disobedient" and "with no way of improving". Many of the parents who belong to families whose characteristics reveal neglect or violence (physical or psychological) have experienced abuse as children and are usually users of alcohol and other drugs.

Families with cases of child sexual abuse show different characteristics from families with episodes of violence or neglect. The former show an exaggerated level of care and protection for the child or adolescent, demonstrating rigid control over social relationships, showing exaggerated possessiveness and jealousy, prohibiting dating relationships and showing permanent distrust. These families often accuse the child or adolescent of seductive or promiscuous behavior, showing a clear reversal of roles, i.e. it is usual for the daughter to play the role of mother in the home (FARINATTI, 1992; FURNISS, 1993; FERRARI, 1997; MARTNS, 1997; CAMINHA, 1999).

The abusive use of alcohol and other drugs, as well as the fact that the parents were subjected to abuse in their childhood are traits commonly found in the families of children subjected to intrafamily violence (FARINATTI, 1992; GUERRA, 1998; CAMINHA, 1999).

Children who are victims of physical or psychological violence, neglect or sexual violence have a low frustration threshold and are economically and emotionally dependent on the adults around them. They are sad, isolated, withdrawn and have low self-esteem. They are usually hyperactive and have aggressive and rebellious behavior. At school, they show learning problems and a constant state of alertness; they are always on the defensive; they are excessively embarrassed; they run away from physical contact; they tend to have suicidal ideas and/or attempts. There may also be constant fatigue, loss or excess of appetite, enuresis and/or encopresis, malnutrition, observable physical injuries, urinary infections, pain or swelling in the genital or anal area, sexually transmitted diseases, age-inappropriate behaviour (seductive or sexualized). They may also have a history of running away or reluctance to return home (WHALEY and WONG, 1989; FARINATTI, 1992; CAMINHA, 1999).

Regarding the exercise of violence, Santos (1998, p. 42) describes the feelings of the abused child:

> Experience shows that the child or adolescent who suffers violence often believes that they are responsible, that they are the cause of their own suffering because they have been disobedient, bad or seductive. They represent themselves as a being who has nothing good inside them, nothing to give, and for this reason they are mistreated or neglected. This belief on the part of the child is usually reinforced by the aggressor himself, who justifies his violence by blaming the victim.

Just as the symptoms and signs of abuse are many and varied, so are the situations and the way in which they are presented. Whether in the form of neglect, physical or sexual violence, or manifested in more or less privileged classes, violence has been pointed out as a reality of our time. Its estimates are frightening, not least because of the alarming rate at which it is growing. I understand that violence against children is a wide-ranging phenomenon, which must be understood from different perspectives and not only from the point of view of the person who suffers it, but also from the point of view of the processes involved in sustaining and maintaining violent actions towards children.

4. SOCIAL EDUCATION

Understanding the importance of education in the current global economic and social climate, and believing that every human being has the right to it and, therefore, to a dignified standard of living, I have tried, through the following reflections, to delve deeper into what social education means for a better future for all of humanity.

According to Zanela (2004, p. 13), "perhaps in the future education will be part of the daily lives of all Brazilians". This idea reflects the concern of many educators, which I share: concern about people's access to education. It also prompts us to question why, then, our education is permeated by neglect and indifference on the part of certain segments.

Individuals are responsible for their own learning, but this doesn't mean that it depends exclusively on them, since I see their educational context as broad, thus requiring the participation of parents, the school itself, the government and society in general, because I understand that education starts from a process of analysis and reflection on reality, in search of the development of autonomy and greater awareness, conceiving of the individual as someone who is critically inserted into history and who is capable of problematizing it and overcoming its limitations, through competent and ethical intervention.

Thus, the goal of every educator should be to prepare the individual to face challenges, to question their reality with a view to transforming it, through experiences that favor their biopsychosocial growth and the construction of Christian values, such as respect, solidarity and justice.

Oliveira (2004, p. 15) emphasizes that in our country today there is a life situation, for large sections of the population, of material, emotional and spiritual poverty and misery in the midst of tremendous wealth and abundance, reflected in the astronomical profits of the banks and telecommunications companies, and the immeasurable and untouchable fortunes of the corrupt.

The possibility of people thinking about this is a threat, and the job of the social educator, I understand, is precisely to encourage people to think about how they are, where they are and what can be changed.

According to Lopez Martin (2000, p. 21), Social Education

"It is, therefore, a type of social intervention, carried out using educational strategies and content, in areas that promote well-being and improve the quality of life, through a series of mechanisms aimed at solving problems of need for marginalized groups, preventing problems for the population in general, guaranteeing a series of rights for a correct community life and, in short, optimizing the processes of socialization."

Reflecting on Social Education thus means corroborating what Lopèz Martin (2000, p. 41) says:

"Transforming reality for a better society, fully developing our commitment to the generalization of the common good becomes the main identity trait of the social educator"; and points out that "energizing cultures, organizing collectives, ensuring the active participation of all citizens, fighting against forms of exclusion and discrimination, defending the universal implementation of human rights or working for the democratic ideals of political tolerance and respect, will be some of the most marked ideological signs.

We live in a society in crisis, not only from an economic point of view, with absolute poverty and high levels of unemployment, but also from a profound crisis of values that leads us to countless problems, such as drug trafficking, prostitution, alcoholism, poor public services and schools, low investment in health, education and preventive actions, crime and a variety of forms of violence against life. The social diagnosis is of homes and communities plagued by family violence, which today is a serious collective health problem.

I understand that violence in family relationships is part of the world of power relations, in which everyone has their share of responsibility, because thinking about intrafamily violence brings us back to the analysis that prior to it, or with it, the state is silent on issues of protection and assistance to families so that they have the necessary conditions to ensure the fundamental rights of children.

I believe that intrafamily violence is multi-causal, that is, it results from the confluence of various aspects; therefore, the dynamics of the violent relationship between parents and children cannot be understood without considering how the conditions surrounding the family affect this relationship. Thus, the history of violent interaction between parents and children is considered an important indicator of the quality of life of these families, since it often covers situations with long-lasting problems, such as poverty, addiction to alcohol and other drugs, and chronic illnesses. According to Cabral (1999), the social costs of domestic violence in Brazil, associated with hospital admissions and absenteeism from work, mean that the Brazilian economy loses

10.5% of its gross domestic product.

It is important to note that violence against children in the family is underpinned by structural violence, involving unequal access to services. Precarious housing conditions, unemployment and the poverty that plagues a large part of the population are factors that, together with the stress they generate, contribute significantly to the increase in the rate of intrafamily violence in our country; however, it should be emphasized that the factors that generate intrafamily violence against children go beyond socioeconomic conditions.

Social inequality in Brazil puts children at risk, as they grow up without dignified survival conditions and with few possibilities for improvement.

I understand that professionals who work with the problem of intrafamily violence from a social education perspective use intervention methods that aim to transform social conditions and reduce stress in families. Short-term interventions include dealing with housing, financial and work problems, providing practical support such as basic childcare and household chores, and expanding and strengthening the family support network. In the long term, the need to work on establishing family protection policies, housing policies, income redistribution and other policies that can guarantee citizenship rights.

Within this perspective of Social Education, it is not enough to deal only with the physical and psychological problems of intra-family violence, but it is necessary to deal with the social violence that underlies the problem of intra-family violence against children.

5. HEALTH EDUCATION

According to Mosquera and Stobaus (1984), Health Education should be aimed at a healthy person, physically, psychologically and socially. The authors understand the person not only as an individual, but also as a representative of a group and a whole. Thus, they emphasize that the health of the person represents the health of the group, and the group represents the health of the institutions. As people have a better level of physical, psychological and social health, societies tend to be fairer, more balanced and more coherent.

Relating the theme of violence to Health Education shows that it is part of a whole that aims to lead to learning better ways of living for one's own performance, enabling the subject to gain greater self-knowledge and also greater knowledge of their environment and community.

As Costa and Lòpez (1986, p. 141) point out, "today, the greatest concern of health educators is how to get people, groups and communities to actually adopt health-facilitating behaviors".

Morais (1995, p. 13) asks "why has our civilization become so violent? Is it still possible to admit that anyone can claim to be healthy in such a sick society?". I believe so, and I also think that health education is an essential part of the practice of any health professional, especially nurses. It's not enough just to recognize that the population has the right to health and the need to make proper use of health services, because this alone is not enough to motivate individuals to change their behavior, since there are socio-economic and political issues that often act as a barrier to healthy behavior among the population.

Most of the time, families that experience violence in their internal dynamics show precarious living conditions, such as a lack of basic hygiene, health, food and housing, among other factors. These are the main manifestations of structural violence, which deeply affects children, placing them in a serious situation of vulnerability and being a source of great suffering for them and their families.

I think that children have different needs from adults and need to be understood and respected as human beings in a peculiar condition of development, as beings with rights and duties, but in accordance with these needs.

It is important to emphasize that the practice of intra-family violence, in its various forms, must be combated, so that violence against children is not naturalized, that it is recognized as a crime and punished by law; in addition, it is a priority to give children an absolute guarantee of access to knowledge of their rights.

Reflecting on the theme of violence in relation to Health Education means realizing that both the individuals who suffer from this problem and many of the professionals in the fields of Education and Health are unaware of the appropriate actions and resources available, not only in terms of intervention plans, but also in terms of preventing the phenomenon.

I therefore believe that Educating for Health is a fundamental element for and in the formation of a better critical awareness among the population, emphasizing participation and co-responsibility for the exercise of full citizenship.

The need to address intrafamily violence through the theme of Health Education is justified since it should promote a greater understanding of the aspects surrounding the problem by professionals, enabling interdisciplinary care that is more suited to the needs of the family and encouraging a more efficient and integrated use of resources. Since the family environment is the child's original context of functioning, if this context cannot be improved, rebuilt, there could be a great risk of destructive or self-destructive behavior appearing, with the prolongation and projection of this type of behavior onto adults in the family, school and society.

It is in this dynamic that a culture of violence is established within the family, which associates violence with social violence, because it is known that children's first forms of interaction can strongly shape their history. To live in an environment surrounded by violence is to leave the child vulnerable to inadequate, bad forms of relationships, which will certainly mark their life. Thus, I believe that the family ends up reproducing, through violence against children, the structural violence to which it is subjected.

It is therefore possible to agree with Muszkat (2002) that families are unprepared to understand, manage and tolerate their own conflicts and end up becoming violent by tradition. Violent homes leave their children with a legacy of violence. I understand that when children begin to live with violence, whether physical or symbolic, either through abuse by adults or by observing violent relationships between these adults, they learn that it is through violence that conflicts are resolved. Violent families therefore produce many more violent people, through the so-called intergenerational cycle of violence. From this perspective, we can see violent children and adults contributing both to the perpetuation of this cycle and to its growth.

6. NURSING EDUCATION

Education is a human activity that is necessary for the existence and functioning of all societies, it is a social and universal phenomenon, according to Libâneo (1994).

I understand that it is through educational action that the social environment influences individuals, and by assimilating and recreating these influences they become capable of establishing an active and transformative relationship in the social environment.

Gadotti (1993) points out that education is considered to be emancipatory when it sets out to create, through its process, a critical conscience, thus instrumentalized to seek transformations. Creating this critical consciousness means integrating the human being into the social context, but not in a passive way, as an object adjusted or accommodated to situations, but as a free, active subject with a creative and renewing capacity.

Eidt, Biehl and Algeri (1998), in their article entitled "Atelier de vivencias: um ambiente propicio a construçà ao cuidado à criança hospitalizada por maus-ratatos" (An environment conducive to the construction of care for children hospitalized for abuse), discusses the learning experienced by the nursing team, concluding that, in the care and monitoring of families who had their children hospitalized due to physical trauma resulting from situations of intra-family violence, nursing care was fragmented, as it excluded educational aspects, considered relevant to the opportunity for individuals to transform their violent behavior.

I believe that the right way to deal with intrafamily violence must be in the field of Education associated with Health, because nurses, when caring for children who have been victims of intrafamily violence, are often faced with the following feelings

of rejection of the guardians of these children; however, I realize that this is not the best course of action, as they also need specialized support and guidance to adopt other patterns of relationship with the child.

Often, the type of relationship between parents and children, which leads to violence, is a reaction by these families to survive in the face of various problems, suffering and social disruption; Therefore, it is essential that nurses, when faced with the reality of intra-family violence, in the process of caring for children, often during a period of prolonged hospitalization, try to understand that if, on the one hand, they find themselves immersed in the problems of families, being affected by these problems, they need to establish a limit between the exercise of technical activities, professional commitment in situations in which they can interfere positively, when they are faced with the powerlessness to change a reality on their own which will only be transformed by the action and investment of the collective, of society as a whole, and also of the individual subjects of intrafamily violence.

The closeness and bonds formed between child, family and team allow relationships to be deepened, making it possible to direct existing conflicts and problems towards less destructive and healthier ways of coping.

In this sense, Jacquard (2002), prefacing the book "The construction of knowledge and citizenship", points out that "the primary function of the entire community, after having fulfilled the conditions of biological survival, is to ensure that each of its members takes advantage of the fabulous power it possesses: to transmute a homo, defined by his genetic heritage, into a man, defined by the bonds he weaves with others."

As nurses unveil the reality of intrafamily violence in the care process, they build up experiences and knowledge, respecting the uniqueness of the situations; in this way, they become critical and responsible for the learning process, shared in parallel with families in situations of intrafamily violence and with other health professionals.

Nursing professionals become more qualified when they come into contact with the phenomenon of intrafamily violence and begin a process of problematizing intervention to change this situation.

Moraes and Eidt (1999) mention the difficulties that professionals, such as nurses, have in dealing with situations of family violence in their day-to-day work, due to their lack of academic preparation. This makes it clear to me that there is a need to include knowledge about intrafamily violence against children in curricula and to provide them with opportunities to take part in workshops such as the ones in this study, in order to develop their potential in relation to the prevention of intrafamily violence and comprehensive health care for children and adolescents in their families.

7. TYPE OF STUDY

This study was characterized as a case study with a qualitative approach. The methodological choice was based on my belief that, in order to understand the reasons, perceptions and possible alternatives for minimizing violence against children, this is the type of study that seemed most appropriate.

As Haguette (1987, p. 63) points out, "qualitative methods emphasize the specificities of a phenomenon in terms of its origins and its reason for being".

According to Pedro (2000, p. 85), another factor that contributed to the choice of qualitative research is that in this study "the interaction between researcher and researched is significant and experiences can be exchanged when the former is not the owner of knowledge and the latter is someone who knows nothing and can allow himself to be invaded in his context". Invaded should be understood here as the researched.

The case study is a type of research that deeply analyzes "something singular, which has value in itself", as Lüdke and André (1986, p.17) point out. These authors also highlight as fundamental characteristics that a case study "aims at discovery, as well as emphasizing interpretation in context, seeking to portray reality in a complete and profound way, using various sources of information, revealing vicarious experience and seeking to represent the different points of view in a given situation".

Stake (1998, p. 15) states that "the qualitative researcher highlights subtle differences, the sequence of events in their context and the globality of personal situations". Case study research is not an investigation of samples; the primary objective is, according to the same author, to understand these selected cases.

The author comments on some criteria that should be used to select cases. One of them is the profitability of what we have learned, which I understand in this context as what we are going to understand; another is the time available to the researcher for the field study and the possibility of access to it and, if possible, the choice of cases that are easy to approach.

This research was therefore concerned with carrying out workshops with guardians aggressors who used violent behavior towards their children, accompanying them and listening to them during their participation in workshops in a public hospital, and after the workshops.

8. THEMATIC AREA

Intrafamily violence is a major cause of injury to children, possible subsequent physical or mental disability and even death in childhood. This phenomenon, as a broad collective health problem, emerges from the internal dynamics of each family, added to external factors such as the socio-economic, political and cultural context in which it is inserted.

Although this is a complex issue, I believe that by getting to know the perceptions of those responsible for the child and the reasons that led them to use violent behavior towards their children, as a way of trying to educate them that is even socially accepted, we also intend to discuss possible alternatives with these families, with a view to a new, healthier approach, in the sense of proposing different forms of relationship with the child throughout the educational process, as proposed by Kaplan and Sadock (1997), Azevedo and Guerra (1989) and Farinatti et al. (1992).

Based on these findings from my reading and my experiences as a nurse and educator, I defined the research topic as follows: *Workshops with aggressive mothers to help change violent behavior.*

With this, I will be able, based on the results of the research, to propose alternative educational actions for those responsible, in relation to the practice of violent behavior towards children, reported as a way of educating, extending this scope to society, to professionals in the areas of Health and Education influential in the process of prevention and or intervention in different levels of intrafamily violence,

9. GUIDING QUESTIONS

How does the perpetrator perceive violence as a form of education?

How does the perpetrator participate in educational workshops?

What does the perpetrator report after the workshop about the change in his child's educational behavior?

What alternatives for educational actions emerged from the workshops and the perceptions of those responsible?

10. FIELD OF STUDY

The research took place in a public university hospital in Porto Alegre.

In 1990, through Federal Law No. 8063, the Statute of the Child and Adolescent came into force, which disseminates the Doctrine of Comprehensive Child Protection, based on the recognition of special and specific rights arising from the peculiar condition of developing people. With regard to professional responsibility in the notification of cases, the Child and Adolescent Statute states in its article 245 (Brasil 1990, p.86) that

"Failure by a doctor, teacher or person in charge of a health care establishment, elementary school, pre-school or nursery school to report to the competent authority any cases of which he or she becomes aware, involving suspicion or confirmation of ill-treatment of a child or adolescent: Penalty fine of three to twenty reference salaries, doubled in the case of repeat offenses."

The hospital therefore has a multi-professional team made up of pediatricians, psychiatrists, social workers, psychologists and nurses, who are assisted by professionals from the Public Prosecutor's Office.

At the same time as reporting cases to the relevant public bodies, such as guardianship councils or the Public Prosecutor's Office, and accompanying children and their families, the team, of which the researcher is a member, opened up spaces for educational workshops, as an alternative methodological proposal for tackling this problem.

11. STUDY PARTICIPANTS

The research participants were five aggressor mothers, responsible for children in situations of physical intrafamily violence, who took part in the ten educational workshops held by members of this program. The number of participants was established according to the criterion of information saturation.

In this study, those responsible for the children who suffered violence were families registered at the hospital, and the sample consisted of five aggressor mothers.

Previously, their medical records were searched in order to obtain sociodemographic information that would help identify the participants in the study (Appendix A).

In order to take part in the study, inclusion and exclusion criteria were adopted. The inclusion criteria were:

- being a parent responsible for a child in a situation of physical intrafamily violence;
- having taken part in the ten workshops offered by the professionals working on the subject at the hospital;
- being the perpetrator of the action of hitting the child;
- voluntarily agreed to take part in the study, following a verbal invitation from the researcher, after having been informed of its objectives.

The exclusion criteria for the study were:

- had emotional, clinical or social alterations that prevented the interviews from being carried out, as well as being drunk or on drugs at the time the instrument was applied;
- refuse to take part in the research;

The profile of these mothers shows that they worked double shifts, outside and inside the home. Most of their paid jobs were as cleaners or housekeepers. The average family income was one minimum wage.

Three families were nuclear, made up of husband, wife and children, and in one family the father was in prison, but the couple remained legally married.

Two of the families were single-parent families with trigerational characteristics, with the maternal grandmother living with the family.

Most of the family members had incomplete primary education; only one mother had completed high school, but incompletely. This mother reported that, after working in the workshops, she had enrolled in a supplementary school to complete high school.

The criteria for inclusion in the workshops were established by considering the profile of motivation and adherence demonstrated during the process of monitoring and treatment in hospital due to the associated physical and psychological abuse and neglect.

Participation in the workshops is seen by the team working with violence as a continuation of the treatment offered by the hospital.

From a systemic point of view, when mothers came to the workshops, they brought their children with them. The invitation to take part in the workshops was extended to fathers, grandparents, uncles and other Significant Carers. All the participants carried out the same activities, although in some workshops the children were separated from the adults and took part in recreational activities promoted by the hospital's Recreation Service.

12. BIOETHICAL CONSIDERATIONS

Ethical principles were safeguarded, as the research was assessed and approved by the hospital's Ethics Committee and by the Research Committee of the UFRGS Faculty of Nursing, as well as protecting the rights of those being researched, taking into account the determinations set out in the norms for health research referred to in Resolution No. 0196, of October 10, 1996, of the National Health Council of the Ministry of Health (BRASIL, 1996) and the ethical issues for nursing research expressed by Polit and Hungler (1995).

The participants who agreed to take part in this research signed a Free and Informed Consent Form (FICF), in which the objectives and implications of their participation were explained, and they were guaranteed confidentiality, anonymity and the possibility of leaving the study at any time.

The ICF identifies that the object of the study is the perceptions of the children's guardians about the reasons that lead them to hit the children as a form of education. As the purpose of the study was to propose future educational actions, throughout the course of the research we sought to improve its investigative and pedagogical function. Thus, in view of the objectives set, the title of this thesis was chosen: *Repercussões de Oficinas para a Educaçao de Responsáveis Aggressores: Interfaces entre Educaçao Social, Educaçao para Saúde e Educaçao em Enfermagem.*

13. DATA COLLECTION

Once the mothers responsible for the children had been selected to take part in the workshops and agreed to take part in the study, the data collection procedures began. Data was collected using three instruments. The first consisted of a semi-structured interview (Appendix B), collected before and during the workshops. This first interview was about *the guardians' perceptions of drumming as a form of education.*

The second instrument was the workshop observation report (Appendix C), which included the guiding questions, and the third was the second semi-structured interview, which took place six months after the workshops (Appendix D).

The interview is a face-to-face meeting between the researcher and the subject, in which the subject and the interviewer share specific information related to the objective of the study in a direct way, with the possibility of interfering and asking for additions. The interview was carried out in the hospital itself, in a place that guaranteed privacy and security, free from risks of intrusion, at a time of the participants' convenience; it was recorded and transcribed immediately afterwards, in accordance with the authorization previously granted by the interviewee.

Observation allowed the researcher to take note of elements that were not explained in the interviews, but happened in the course of the research.

The observations took place during the workshop meetings.

14. CONTEXT FOR THE WORKSHOPS

In order to better characterize these workshops, which became the environment for collecting data for this research, it was considered essential to describe the context in which they took place.

Preventing situations of violence is also an educational requirement, as well as a social and legal one; therefore, it is essential that this takes place in an interactive, reflective and critical environment. This requires the participation of a multidisciplinary team to provide support and specific guidance.

Thus, the workshops were a space for multidisciplinary action, in an educational process with aggressor mothers who had experienced situations of violence that integrated my beliefs, values and attitudes, as a nurse and researcher, with the studies carried out in the Doctorate Course of the Postgraduate Program in Education at PUC.

The workshops were held with the general aim of developing an interdisciplinary care and educational process with children and their families and/or caregivers who have experienced situations of intrafamily violence at the hospital.

The workshops had the following specific objectives: To provide guidance on biopsychosocial health care, human rights, citizenship and legislation, combining these topics with others of interest to them.

To provide aggressors with learning strategies to improve their ability to care for the child.

Motivate participants to raise awareness and form critical judgments about intrafamily violence, with the aim of improving the quality of life for themselves and their families.

Strengthening family ties in order to reduce or eradicate the problem of violence diagnosed.

To provide support for positive changes in family relationships. Prevent recurrences of violence against children.

To train the families who attended the workshops to become multipliers of the child protection ideology in their communities.

The workshops also made it possible to train undergraduate students in Nursing, Psychology and Social Work to act as multipliers in the prevention, diagnosis and treatment of children and family members in situations of intrafamily violence.

In methodological terms, the workshop had the characteristics of an educational group, and used the pedagogical option of problematization (BORDENAVE, 1983), taking into account that what was desired was the transformation of the reality of intra-family violence based on modifying the behavior of the aggressor mothers through their own observations and perceptions of the reality of violence that they lived in the family environment or provided for their children.

The participants were encouraged to detect real problems and seek original and creative solutions. According to Bourdenave (1983), this pedagogy does not separate individual transformation from social transformation, which develops in group situations.

The whole process of the workshops emerged from the experiences and relationships of the group members in order to create subsidies that would eliminate the practice of any form of violence against children, making it possible to form healthier relationships within the family.

According to the Ministry of I lealth (1997), in the workshops, the educational process through participation took place through a process of theorizing from practice, not as a substitution for theoretical content, but as a systematic, orderly, progressive process, at the pace of the participants, allowing them to discover the theoretical elements through the techniques and to gradually deepen them, according to the level of progress of the group.

Through theory, the workshops were a guide to transformative practice.

The process of theorizing allowed everyday life to be placed - the immediate, the individual and the partial - within the social, the collective, the historical and the structural.

The participatory techniques developed in the workshops provided a learning process through which it was possible to develop a collective process of discussion and reflection that allowed individual knowledge to be collectivized in a way that boosted the knowledge of the other participants, made it possible to develop a common educational reflection experience and enabled the collective creation of knowledge, in the elaboration of which all the individuals took part.

In order to read the reality and identify the key points of the problems experienced by the mothers taking part in the study, as well as to understand the phenomenon and to find the necessary solutions that are feasible and applicable, we used theoretical and legal support based on the rights of children and adolescents, biopsychosocial and health needs, human rights, citizenship, gender, parental bonds, prevention of physical trauma in children, self-esteem, concepts of physical, psychological and sexual violence, neglect and drug abuse30, among others, according to the themes that emerged and were of interest to the participants.

The proposed intervention was carried out by a multi-professional team made up of two nurses, two social workers, a pediatrician, a recreationist, a psychologist, a public prosecutor and interns from the nursing, psychology and social work departments.

In all the activities, there was always a nursing, psychology and/or social work trainee observing the activity in order to record the dynamics and results of the workshops.

The workshops were also held in the hospital itself, seeking to expand the care strategies that the mothers received, in addition to the care already offered by the institution, making other care alternatives possible, as this type of group work made it possible to share similar experiences among the families of caregivers with a history of family violence.

The issues addressed in the workshops emerged from the facilitators' experiences and their knowledge of the problem of violence in these families. They focused on the Statute of the Child and Adolescent, as well as questions about citizenship, the child's stage of growth and development, housing conditions, basic hygiene and health habits, among others. This is justified by the fact that these families and/or caregivers were unaware of their rights as citizens, of the present and future psychosocial consequences and of the fact that intra-family violence is illegal.

The work of the workshops always included spaces to deal with issues that were brought up by the participants themselves. This contributed to reflection and criticism, facilitated the exchange of experiences, constituting an educational group, integrated with the interdisciplinary team, providing support and specific guidance. The presence of play and games in this context facilitated reorganization and family ties, creating a space for problem solving.

I believe that the workshops we held provided new support for interdisciplinary care, which is necessary in these circumstances, as we worked on the multidimensionality of its causes and consequences. I therefore believe that future workshops will provide opportunities to build new knowledge, taking into account care processes, in order to help create new prevention strategies that are relevant to the situation of this group. At the same time, it enabled the mutual growth of the professionals involved in the process of caring, teaching and learning.

Therefore, the development of these activities, with the help of the team members, makes the workshops a new possibility for a methodological-assistance-educational approach, broadening the way of tackling the issue of intrafamily violence.

In order to cover all the abused mothers referred to us and also to include their family members, it was necessary to divide the participants into two groups, taking care to ensure that the same professionals ran each workshop for both groups.

The workshops were planned to take place in the afternoon, in ten fortnightly meetings for each group, between November 2002 and July 2004, lasting one hour and thirty minutes each.

The scheduled time was from 2pm to 4.30pm on Wednesdays, in order to make it easier for participants to get away from home and work.

The venue for the workshops was a room attached to the hospital, which allowed the group access and privacy.

Ethical principles were respected in an attempt to protect the individual rights of the aggressor participants, taking into account the aspects pointed out by Goldim (2000).

The aim of the workshops was explained, giving participants the option of taking part and joining the group, as well as the guarantee of the conventional individual and family care that they have been receiving systematically in the treatment of intrafamily violence at the hospital, even if they refused to take part.

15. O PROCESS EXPERIENCED IN THE WORKSHOPS

Although the multi-professional team had planned the techniques and objectives for each workshop in advance, because we already knew the reasons and difficulties that led to the referrals of these abuser mothers, there was no systematic sequential prediction of the techniques, except for the first and last two workshops. This was because the course of each meeting made it possible to identify the next most appropriate approach to be developed.

Thus, at the end of each workshop, in a thirty-minute period, the professionals participating in the team analyzed the realities and the main problems brought up, as well as intervention alternatives for possible solutions.

In order to provide a warm welcome and establish bonds between the participants, their families and the team, at the end of each workshop there was an integration in the form of a collective snack offered by the team.

Below are the ten workshops we ran with the mothers taking part in the research and their families.

1ª WORKSHOP CONSTELLATION OF SYMBOLS: THIS IS ME

The aim of the first day was to identify all the participants, discuss the proposed objectives of the workshops, and combine and establish the dynamics for running them.

The meeting had the function of integrating the group and establishing a kind of work contract. This workshop is described in full in Appendix E.

The first meeting was attended by two nurses, a pediatrician, a public prosecutor, a recreationist, a social worker, two psychology trainees, two nursing trainees, five mothers, a grandmother and eight children.

It's worth noting that, in this first meeting, people used the entire workshop to tell us how their families were made up and describe their daily lives, the difficulties in family relationships, especially between the couple, with their children, as well as the problems in their own homes, in relation to the many crises they faced in order to survive, such as drug use, the difficulty of maintaining authority, the division of responsibilities between parents, among others.

Subject A *"People's lives aren't easy, there are so many problems. There are days when you think you're going to go mad".*

Subject B "I'm like all of you here in the group, I hit the kids, but I know I shouldn't, sometimes they end up being hit for things that have nothing to do with them, it's us who lose our temper over something, but it's also so much to deal with. My brother makes everyone's life hell with his drug problem"

Subject C *"I find myself very much on my own to cope with everything. It's true that from time to time my mother helps me in any way she can, but her money is also a pittance, it's not even enough for her, in reality I'm the only one who has to provide for the children".*

Subject D *"The biggest problem I see at home is that as well as the fights with the children, there are my problems with my husband. The children see us fighting, they know we're not well and they repeat what they see of us. Children learn a lot from watching adults, they end up imitating them without even meaning to".*

Subject E *"I thought that when I was pregnant everything would be different. Everyone was going to do my bidding, I was going to be pampered by my mother, but no, nothing has changed."*

From the reports extracted from the first meeting, I was able to infer that the people in the group had similar life situations: they were families in crisis, with all kinds of family, emotional, economic and social difficulties.

In the evaluation of this first meeting, one of the psychology trainees described the activity as a great catharsis, in other words, there was a space for the participants to verbally and emotionally externalize their feelings about life.

In this workshop, a process of exchanging emotions, suffering and learning began. The interaction between family members and the team made it possible to unveil intrafamily violence.

The professionals intervened to enable the participants to freely state their perceptions of the problem they were experiencing in the family, a reality of violence that was common to the group's participants. The team's intervention provided motivation and relaxation for the next activities.

In this sense, it corroborates the idea of Minayo and Assis (1993) when they state that violence is a complex and dynamic biopsychosocial phenomenon, and its space of creation and development is life in society.

2ª WORKSHOP: DRAWING AND EXPLAINING MY WORLD.

The aim of this workshop was to exchange information between the members of the group so that they could get to know each other better and realize the common reality of intrafamily violence that surrounded them.

Each participant made a free drawing and then told the story of each family's life.

The two nurses, the pediatrician, the public prosecutor, the recreationist, a social worker, the two psychology trainees, the two nursing trainees, a social work trainee, five mothers, a grandmother and an aunt took part in this second meeting. The children did not take part in this workshop.

Subject *A "At home it's all about shouting. My husband shouts at me, at the children, and I shout at them too. When I drew the family, I saw that everything is the same for us. It's all just one fight."*

Subject B *"I was hit a lot when I was a child, I can't even compare the way my mother was with me with the way I am with my son, I was hit and sometimes I didn't even know why. My son at least always knows the reason when I hit him, and sometimes it feels like he's asking to be hit*[j,].

Subject C *"It's just like I drew it with strong colors, there's nothing light in my life. It's all heavy, difficult, think of me with two children, pregnant with my third and without the support of their father".*

Subject D *"I keep thinking about what the family I work for is like every day and what mine is like. They're so different, my bosses get on super well, they're always kissing, hugging, and my husband and I just fight. Their children that I look after are calm, polite, and mine are so artistic, so lawless".*

Subject *E "I don't even like to stop to think about what my life is like, because I think it's all bad, it's all crap, my daughters have nothing, in fact, they have the things that others give them, even to eat we depend on others. That's not life.*

This meeting revealed, through the drawings and their interpretation by the speeches, the multiple forms of social exclusion, socio-economic inequalities, the abuse of power by adults over children, the different forms of physical and emotional violence and neglect exercised in families.

During the evaluation, the team noticed that many of the participants' behaviors stemmed from similar situations they had experienced in childhood, and so the intervention explained the importance of them making a commitment to new ways of relating to the child. As an example of the intervention that took place in this workshop, the nurse proposed a task for each participant to carry out over the course of the week. The mothers should try to talk to the children to avoid hitting them and, if talking didn't help to stop the inappropriate behavior, the mothers should take the child on their lap and hold them tightly. Everyone agreed to carry out the proposed activity.

3ª MAGIC BOX WORKSHOP: SELF-IMAGE AND SELF-IMPROVEMENT. WHO ARE WE?

This meeting aimed to explore each participant's concept of themselves, as well as encouraging reflection on the healthy aspects of the participants and the desire to change the aspects that hindered healthy living.

By opening the lid of a box lined with gift paper, the participant saw themselves in a mirror glued to the inside of the box, describing what they liked and disliked about what they saw.

Taking part in this third meeting were the two nurses, the two psychology trainees, a nursing trainee, the public prosecutor, the recreationalist, a social worker, five mothers, a grandmother and an aunt.

The children did not take part in this activity.

Subject A *"Looking at my face I see how much has changed over time, I put on a lot of weight during my last pregnancy, my body isn't that of a beautiful woman".*

Subject B *"I prefer to see myself as I am today than when I was a child. I was an ugly child, too skinny'*

Subject C *"When I look at myself I see how much I've been through in this life. Sometimes I can't believe I've managed to overcome everything, I don't mean everything, but I've overcome a lot of things, a lot of sadness that's been left behind.*

Subject D *"I don't like looking in the mirror. I don't think I'm pretty. I wish I could take care of myself a lot, I'd fill myself up with creams, make-up, these rich woman things, so I wouldn't look ugly, old. I know I look much older than I really am"*

Subject E *"I don't know, it's so weird to look in the mirror and tell other people what you see. I don't like talking about myself, I'm ashamed, sometimes I even feel angry with myself".*

The team intervened through the participants' accounts of the image reflected in the mirror, emphasizing the importance of having moments to look inside ourselves, how we see ourselves as a person in the world, in our family.

It also made it possible to evaluate the importance of exercising our roles as women, mothers, wives and partners, enabling a better understanding of the factors that bother and interfere with self-esteem.

The team worked to encourage participants to accept their own bodies, understanding that ideals of beauty were imposed by culture, that society proposes stereotypes, rigid models of beauty. People start chasing these models, which are usually associated with success, power and social acceptance.

The activity sought to demonstrate the benefits of acquiring a positive body image, as this interferes with the ability to give and receive affection, in the way each person perceives themselves and others. The work highlighted the importance of each person liking themselves and understanding their body, and there were even discussions about how to look after it properly, not least because the body functions as an instrument of interpersonal communication, in which body care reveals the self-esteem that each person has. This is dynamic, perceptible from an understanding of one's sense of identity, personal characteristics, self-worth, achievements and relationships.

4ª STOP WORKSHOP! FREEZING THE SCENE AND MAKING A NEW MOVIE!

The aim of this workshop was to relativize the roles played by parents and children, making it possible to understand the functions and dynamics of the family through the feelings expressed. The game of freezing the scene was used to encourage the overcoming of violent practices and to project different ways of acting in the face of the problems that had arisen.

The team's intervention made it possible for the group to receive guidance and discuss impulse control in physical violence, reporting their difficulties, especially in relation to the child.

This workshop was carried out through the dramatization of a scene from each family, with parents and children exchanging roles, making it possible, in these playful experiences, to review their feelings or discover new ones, in order to discover another way of relating to the child.

The dynamics of the workshop made it possible to review situations of interaction between mothers and their children, pointing out new ways of imposing affective and firm limits on children that did not involve the use of physical violence.

The two nurses, the two psychology interns, a nursing intern, the public prosecutor, the recreationist, a social worker, the pediatrician, a social work intern, five mothers, a father, a grandmother, an aunt and eight children took part in this fourth meeting.

5ª WORKSHOP PLAYING, NOT FIGHTING, WE UNDERSTAND EACH OTHER!

The aim of this workshop was to provide supervised interaction between the children and their mothers.

By proposing playtime in the playground between mothers and their children, the professionals were able to observe and participate in the appropriate handling of the children's demands and the corresponding actions by the mothers. The aggressors' guardians reflected, exchanged ideas and made a commitment to real changes in behavior, which are understood as gradual possibilities.

This workshop was also known by the professionals in the care group as the practice of sensitive listening. The team intervened so that the parents would be aware of, and develop patience and tolerance for, the child's attitudes, which are typical of their stage of growth and development.

The group reflected on the importance of a respectful way of relating to the child, because children learn and internalize patterns of future behaviour from adult attitudes, just as they often act in the present to imitate attitudes and behaviours seen in their parents and caregivers.

The fifth meeting was attended by two nurses, two psychology trainees, a nursing trainee, the public prosecutor, the recreationist, a social worker, the pediatrician, a social work trainee, five mothers, a father, a grandmother, an aunt, a neighbor and ten children.

6ª COLORFUL AND BORDERLESS IMAGINATION WORKSHOP. TELLING CHILDREN'S STORIES.

The aim of this meeting was to stimulate emotional bonds through the living library, i.e. the reading of children's books. This was done by each participant who was responsible for the aggressor. It's worth noting that, in our workshops, the aggressors were made up entirely of the children's mothers.

The team's intervention was to facilitate the experience of pleasurable relationships.

Reading a children's story involves sharing emotions and discoveries that strengthen the emotional bond between child and caregiver.

By reading the stories presented through examples, the team came up with ideas about the importance of working with real values, such as solidarity, respect for differences, friendship and patience, providing the child with subsidies for acquiring positive attitudes throughout life, in the different environments in which they live, such as the family and the school.

Taking part in this sixth meeting were two nurses, two psychology trainees, a nursing trainee, the public prosecutor, the recreationist, a social worker, the pediatrician, a social work trainee, five mothers, a father, a grandmother, an aunt and eight children.

7ª CAUTION WORKSHOP! DANGER LIVES HERE TOO

The aim of this workshop was to prevent domestic accidents. Each participant first reported on a domestic accident they had experienced. Based on the accounts, there was a debate about the situations that caused the accidents and how they could have been avoided, highlighting any involvement related to negligence and violence.

The nurse talked about the growth and development of a child, the activities that each age group performs, the possible causes of accidents related to each age group of their children and how to prevent accidents at each stage of the child's development and growth.

After the dialog, a game was played with the participation of each responsible person to detect fourteen possible causes of accidents in a kitchen with children and ten possible causes of accidents in the yard of a house with children.

The team's intervention was aimed at preventing neglect related to the occurrence of domestic accidents, extending the need for child protection to other situations beyond the home.

The team's work signaled to the participants the possibility of adequate information on how to prevent potential risk situations for domestic accidents, given that the group was generally unaware of situations of individual and family vulnerability and the household risks associated with these occurrences.

The seventh meeting was attended by a nurse, a psychology trainee, two nursing trainees, the public prosecutor, the recreationist, a social worker, the pediatrician, a social work trainee, five mothers, a father, a grandmother and an aunt. The children did not take part in this activity.

8ª WORKSHOP A WAY OF BEING HEALTHY

The aim of this workshop was to provide guidance on hygiene, education and health habits, nutrition, vaccinations, the importance of supervision and health checks according to age, health needs and problems, among other things. Using clippings from magazines and newspapers, the group put together a panel identifying the healthy and vulnerable aspects of each family, and discussed their lifestyle habits, including attendance at health services. In the presentation of the work, each participant explained the reason for the figures they had chosen, describing their current reality and projecting changes for the future.

The team intervened to help the group experience the sense of responsibility involved in motherhood and caring for children.

The work carried out made it possible to discuss aspects of beliefs, values, traditions and attitudes towards health care, and also promoted reflection on the difficulties of seeking health resources for oneself and one's family, as well as alternatives to minimize this problem.

The two nurses, two psychology trainees, two nursing trainees, the public prosecutor, the recreationist, a social worker, the pediatrician, a social work trainee, five mothers, a father, a grandmother and an aunt took part in this eighth meeting. The children did not take part in this activity.

9ª WORKSHOP REDESIGNING LIFE

This workshop aimed to apply networking to the full protection of children's rights through a game that linked the network of institutions and the articles included in the Statute of the Child and Adolescent. The group also worked on gender and citizenship.

The group began with the social worker explaining the importance of working with the rights of children and adolescents in accordance with the ECA. She then showed a board with the rights of children and adolescents drawn on it and each participant in the group read out one of the rights, reflecting, along with the public prosecutor, on what they saw as their own meaning and responsibility.

The team's intervention enabled them to rethink and plan new attitudes and take responsibility for them, including them in their family life project. The workshop sought to reflect on the educational attitudes adopted on a daily basis.

The team's work questioned the positions that men and women occupy in society and pointed out the importance of equal rights under the Brazilian Constitution.

The ninth meeting was attended by two nurses, two psychology interns, two nursing interns, the public prosecutor, the recreationist, a social worker, the pediatrician, a social work intern, five mothers, a grandmother, an aunt, a neighbor and eight children.

10th WORKSHOP THE PRECIOUS GIFT

The aim of this workshop was to encourage participants to reflect on what they should know and what they can do to transform aggressive attitudes into interactive attitudes of care and protection.

Each child painted their hand on a large T-shirt, and each mother painted her hand on a smaller T-shirt; after the paint dried, the T-shirts were exchanged between mother and child and worn by the participants.

The team's intervention, by encouraging the personalized construction of each T-shirt, sought to expand the meaning of awareness, symbolized by the drawing of the hands that represented the collective construction of a new reality, since previously the hands were representative of something threatening, causing pain and suffering.

The exchange of the gift represented the experience of affection, and the drawings of the hands indicated the construction of a new reality, built together, without violence.

Taking part in this tenth meeting were two nurses, two psychology trainees, two nursing trainees, the public prosecutor, the recreationist, a social worker, the pediatrician, a social work trainee, two volunteer plastic artists, five mothers, a grandmother, an aunt and eight other children.

This was the final meeting of the workshops. After handing out the T-shirts and exchanging them between mother and son, the participants evaluated the work of the workshops.

All the comments highlighted the importance of having a space where people could be heard and respected. One of the mothers reported that she had discovered a new way of relating to her children, that the children were calmer and that she was liking herself better, pointing out that she was finding it essential to take care of herself and that this was only possible through the workshops, as she had learned important things to improve her life,

According to a young teenager who recently had a baby during the workshops, she cried and said that her bond with her mother had improved a lot, and that she felt more capable of looking after the baby that had been born, unlike her other child, because when she had her first child she felt very alone, scared and unprepared to be a mother. She believes that the workshops served to show her how to be a good mother, as well as bringing her family closer together.

Three mothers reported the importance of the work done to clarify important doubts they had about the children's behavior and how best to act with their children.

One aunt emphasized that the workshops were not only worthwhile for improving the lives of the children, but also for the whole family, who gained from the work done with the mothers and children.

One grandmother said it was important for the workshops to continue because it was something different and very good that had happened in her life.

DISCOVERIES ALONG THE WAY IN THE WORKSHOPS

After each workshop, the group of professionals evaluated and planned a new meeting. All the workshops were developed and analyzed by the professionals, but the participants' experiences and reports were used as a starting point for trying to eradicate violent behavior and for the necessary transformations.

The situations recorded here show the experience of a multi-professional group that sought to develop workshop work with

children who are victims of domestic violence and their families, which we called the Child Violence Prevention Assistance Group (GAP). The group sought to reflect on the cycle of violence installed in the families that took part in the workshops, and to break it by promoting awareness and critical judgment about violence against children, together with the perpetrators, with the aim of improving the quality of relationships for everyone involved.

The workshops held by the multi-professional team were a complement to the care provided to children in the hospital and were an important educational methodological alternative in dealing with intrafamily violence. The quality of the results was influenced by the bringing together of professionals from different areas who share years of experience in combating violence against children.

The workshops were an activity that needs to be publicized and expanded, as they enabled a great deal of exchange, not only from the point of view of professional knowledge, but also affective knowledge, which allowed each of the participants to teach and learn at the same time.

I believe that there is a pressing need to share ideas and experiences among professionals who work with the phenomenon of intrafamily violence in order to discover new ways of dealing with the situation.

In this sense, I corroborate Vieira and Volquind's (2002) idea that workshops create real situations of participation, in which experiences are socialized and innovative actions are planned, executed and evaluated.

The group work developed in the workshops was important because it allowed a broad approach to violence, corresponding to preventive and humanized work, from an interdisciplinary and intersectoral perspective. Through reflection activities linked to the significant aspects of the reality experienced, the acquisition of knowledge and attitudes for solving or minimizing the problem of intrafamily violence was awakened.

The group's interaction implied emotional support, the strengthening of psychological interactions, frank communication, commitment and responsibility for the group's decisions and actions, as well as effective participation and the formation of individuals' critical awareness.

I agree with Minayo and Assis (1993, p. 59) when they point out that "there is a consensus today that any action to overcome violence requires intersectoral, interdisciplinary, multi-professional coordination with civil society and community organizations that campaign for rights and citizenship".

The workshops were a type of action that provided individuals with the opportunity to reflect on the reality they were experiencing, creating a basis for making changes. It was a space for acquiring new knowledge through the exchange of experiences in groups.

The participants in the workshops had a common reality, which was intra-family violence, so they took on the shared responsibility of changing their attitude towards violent behavior towards children, looking for another way of dealing with this real problem in their lives. In this way, as Cubers (1989, p. 3) points out, "the workshop is a time and space for learning; an active process of reciprocal transformation between subject and object; a path with alternatives".

16. DATA ANALYSIS

After collecting the data, the interviews and workshop observation reports were analyzed using the Content Analysis technique proposed by Bardin (2000), which is used in qualitative research and in various sectors of the human sciences. This research technique aims to formulate, from the data, possible reproducible and valid inferences that can be used in the context under examination.

Bardin (2004, p. 42) defines the method of Content Analysis as

> [...I a set of techniques for analyzing communications, aiming to obtain, through systematic and objective procedures for describing the content of messages, quantitative or non-quantitative indicators that allow the inference of knowledge about the conditions of production/reception (inferred variables) of these messages.

The significance of content analysis is related to the improvement of the technique, which made it possible to interpret sacred texts, with the possibility of uncovering the symbolic meaning of religious acts and the interpretation of literary texts. From the 1950s-60s onwards, this technique began to be used on a large scale as a means of analyzing mass communications. The inferences or logical deductions from this practice can answer two types of production or reception questions.

In this study, the technique was concerned with the question of production, i.e. the possible causes or antecedents of a message, which include the characteristics and origins of the sender and the context; in particular, it investigated the aggressor mothers responsible for the children in situations of domestic violence who took part in the ten workshops. The technique was systematized into three distinct chronological stages: pre-analysis, the material exploration phase and the treatment, inference and interpretation of the data.

In the pre-analysis, supported by the theoretical framework, I first carried out a floating reading of all the subjects' interviews, as well as using elements from the identification forms and partial workshop reports to complement the study. It should be noted that each subject, at this stage, was coded with the letter S (subject) and a corresponding number (1,2,3,4 and 5). In order to comply with the rule of exhaustiveness, i.e. the rules in which you can't leave out any of the elements, I did several readings of all the interviews with each of the five subjects interviewed before and after the workshops. With regard to the rule of representativeness, which concerns sampling in this type of research, I considered that the testimonies of the five subjects and the workshop observation report were representative elements for this investigation. With regard to the homogeneity rule of this type of analysis, all the information was obtained in the same way, i.e. all the subjects were interviewed and observed in the same way by the researcher.

After the pre-analysis, in the material exploration phase, the second phase of the method, which can take place simultaneously with the pre-analysis, the data obtained was coded "in order to reach the core of understanding the text", according to Minayo (1992, p.210). Therefore, I used elements from the identification forms and partial workshop reports to complement the data, thus breaking down the collected material, grouping expressions, ideas, speeches and behaviors, classifying them into units of meaning, using specific coding. (S pre and the number indicate the subject interviewed before the workshop and the unit of meaning corresponding to that interview, while S post and the number indicate the subject interviewed after the workshop and the corresponding unit of meaning). This made it possible to draw up the categories and sub-categories of this study. The criterion for cutting out the units of meaning in this investigation was thematic, involving capturing the meaning of the information recorded by the researcher.

In the third phase, i.e. the treatment, inference and interpretation of the results based on the description of each category, I presented the results of this study, interpreting the data with the help of the authors used in the Theoretical Framework, my experiences and the experiences of the subjects, using elements from the identification forms and the partial reports of the workshops to complement the data collected in the interviews. Thus, according to Santos (1996), a new theoretical perspective emerged as the study's objectives were met.

Based on the analysis of the statements of the perpetrators, two dimensions of this study were formed: the first dimension is the pre-workshop, and the second dimension is the post-workshop, shown in Table 1.

DIMENSION	CATEGORIES	SUBCATEGORIES
Pre-Workshop	Conceptions of education	Related to family history
		Meaning of aggressive action
		Doubts and uncertainties about how to educate
		The way of educating correlates with the child's level of

		development
	Forms of education in practice	From dialogue to shouting
		Intimidation for corporal punishment
		Physical Aspects
		Psychological aspects
	Motives triggering the violent act	Psychosocial characteristics of children
		Psychosocial characteristics of adults
		Fights between brothers
		Maintaining power/authority
		Family dynamics
	Family history	Past/current family history
		Family intervention in the face of violence
		Awakening to the option of professional help
Post-workshop	Experiencing the workshops	The meaning of participation
		The acquisition of knowledge
	Repercussions of the workshops	Pathways to family resilience
		Family and social life
		Preventive aspects
		Suggestions

17. FIRST DIMENSION: PRE-WORKSHOPS

The first dimension of the study presents four categories: the conceptions of how to educate, the forms of education in practice, the reasons for the violent act and the family's trajectory, which emerged from the testimonies collected before the workshops were held.

Category: Conceptions of education

The first category of this study deals with the perpetrators' conceptions of how to educate, which emerged from the interviews with the participants before the workshops took place.

Based on these conceptions, it was possible to obtain four subcategories (shown in Table 1) which allow us to broaden the characterization of the phenomenon under study: related to family history; the meaning of action; doubts and uncertainties about the way of educating; and the way of educating correlated with the child's level of development.

Chart 1- Conceptions of how to educate and their subcategories

Category	Subcategory
lConceptions on how to educate	1.1 Related to family history
	1.2 Meaning of aggressive action
	1.3 Doubts and uncertainties about how to educate
	1.4 Form of education correlates with the child's level of development

Source: Interviews with perpetrators before taking part in the workshops (2005).

1.1 Subcategory related to family history

The subjects' conceptions of the use of violence against children in everyday life can be seen in the statements collected.

As subject D pre 1 said, *"the way I know how to educate children, the original way, which we know and were brought up with, is: you're a nuisance, you're a stick. Didn't obey? Stick. It's all about slapping, shouting and hitting. That's the reality.*

Through the accounts of the aggressors' guardians, I can see that their conceptions of how to educate are linked to family history and tradition, in other words, the use of physical punishment is often adopted by these adults as an internalized way of preventing a certain type of behaviour from the child.

Therefore, this practice emerged and was learned from their own childhood experiences. The use of physical force, i.e. hitting children, is seen in many families as a way for parents to exercise discipline.

This statement is in line with what Neder (1994) says, when he points out that discipline was a fundamental characteristic of the educational process for a long time and that families used countless experiences of physical aggression to achieve it. Spanking children has therefore been part of family education and the pedagogical methods used by families to discipline them.

Subject A pre 10's statement also suggests that the ways in which children are brought up are related to her own childhood experience, as she said they were *"the same as the* way *I was brought up. My mother used to hit me and today I hit my children too".*

Through this testimony, I can see the important role that the family plays, because the practice of using violence against children to educate them is culturally sustained, in other words, it makes the family an opportune space for the use of violence.

Briggs (2002) emphasizes that the discrepancy between the value we place on children, on the one hand, and our inability to provide parents with specific training for their task, on the other, seems to be based on the assumption that a human being should know how to raise another human being; however, the fact that someone becomes a parent does not automatically give them the knowledge and ability to raise children satisfactorily.

Thus, I believe that, through the power relationship between parents and children, there is a clear link between subjection to the form of discipline that often justifies the use of aggression to any degree of violence and the use of violence as a means to an end, because violence is learned in the family of origin of adults and assimilated as a form of education.

Brazelton and Sparrow (2004) warn that parents who were brought up with corporal punishment tend to maintain this tradition in relation to their children. This behavior is often due to a sense of loyalty to their parents and their culture, a sense of duty that leads them to continue their parental obligation, or a lack of other alternatives.

Before choosing how to discipline a child, adults need to be aware of the influence of their personal history, i.e. the way they were disciplined by their parents, because, as parents, there is a tendency for them to adopt the same patterns they were brought up with in childhood or to act completely differently from the way they were brought up. Some parents feel secure in their ability to reproduce the disciplinary traditions of their family, and others have the desire to be different parents from their own; however, most adults use the model they were brought up on to discipline their own children.

Amen (2005) emphasizes that there are many factors involved in raising children and that the aim of effective education is to find the best fit between parents and children, which also means adapting one's personality to the characteristics of the child, given the environment in which they both find themselves.

In this section, it became clear that the educational basis of mothers' disciplinary practices with their children, through physical punishment, came from their own childhood experiences in their family of origin.

1.2 Subcategory the meaning of aggressive action

The words of the perpetrators reveal their lack of understanding of the essential meaning of aggressive action.

Subject B pre 26 said that *"spanking and beating are very different things. Spanking for me is you taking the child and hanging them, throwing them against the wall, stepping on them, hurting them, hitting is you taking a strap or slipper and hitting them on the legs, usually hitting them on the buttocks, because the child doesn't feel it as much".*

The deponent stratifies the acts expressed into different levels of violation of the child's physical integrity, even clarifying the possibility of a pre-determined choice to hit the child on the "ass" in order not to inflict so much pain.

The impression one gets from analyzing the above statement is that the use of violence as a way of educating is not considered in practice to be a violation of children's rights. The act of hitting a child does not mean aggression; on the contrary, hitting is a trivialized and unappreciated strategy.

However, Article 17 of the Statute of the Child and Adolescent (ECA) states that "the right to respect consists of the inviolability of the physical, psychological and moral integrity of children and adolescents [...]".

Subject E pre 1 brought his own meaning to educational action when he said: *"for me*, education *is punishment or beating"*.

I can see from his speech that the meaning he attributes to educating is that of punishment and suffering in both its psychological and physical dimensions, in a unilateral process of adult power and restriction of the rights and autonomy of children and adolescents.

Let's remember Amen (2005), who emphasizes that all parents make mistakes and, no matter how well they do, they will always make some mistakes, but many of them could be avoided if they were well guided and had the chance to reflect on their paternal and maternal role.

I notice that mothers don't contextualize themselves with new educational approaches that exclude the process of hitting children. As a result, they perpetuate acts of discipline that condone physical aggression.

Grünspun clarifies this inadequate context of educating by recalling that, until a few years ago, it was accepted for children to be beaten, which meant educating them (in TIBA, 2002).

1.3 Subcategory Doubts and Uncertainties about how to educate

This subcategory brings together the strategies mentioned by the participants that are used to educate children, but under conditions of doubt and uncertainty about how to educate appropriately; that is, they present ambivalences that show they are between using dialog or corporal punishment.

Subject C pre 1 said: "You have to talk, give limits and punishment. Put them in punishment and let them cry".

I believe that the way in which each adult acts in relation to educating the child is a social construction that varies according to each society and is influenced by different factors, such as the historical, economic and cultural period.

Subject B pre 6's statement illustrated*: "I have doubts. I have a two-year-old son,* *he's impossible. I don't know what to do, if I hit him it won't solve much either. I don't even know anymore, I don't know how to act, I don't know how to educate him properly".*

With constant hesitations in the process of educating a two-year-old, which corresponds to being at an age when children are explorers, curious about everything around them, this mother reveals that the practice of hitting her child doesn't bring the expected educational results; however, she hesitates on how to act differently.

I understand that there are currently a variety of ways of bringing up a child, different strategies are used by families and, most of the time, adults find it difficult to put into practice the most appropriate way of bringing up a child, not feeling satisfactorily prepared to act with the child.

Omer (2002) emphasizes that parental presence contrasts profoundly with authority based on violence, as far as the dignity of the child is concerned. Parental presence is the opposite of tyrannical authority, whose strength comes from punishment and aggression.

The discipline that an adult imposes on a child is a reflection of social values, because, as parents, adults will be held responsible for the child's behavior, so, in a society made up of different cultures like ours, parents need to reflect and understand that disciplinary practices are determined by culture and follow the values and traditions of that culture.

In this sense, Grunspun, in his preface to the book "Quem ama educa" (Who loves educates) (TIBA, 2002), says that, in the name of education, spanking, belting, slapping, shoeing, biting, ear-pulling and hair-pulling were valid. At school, it was worth the rod, the spanking, kneeling on the corn. When a child complained, their mother or father would say it was because they deserved to be spanked.

The following analysis of subject A pre 39's statement suggested that the way she sees fit is dialogue, but when this mother needs to put education into practice, she hits instead of talking. "When I have to talk to my children, there's no point in me hitting them".

Another statement that exemplified the difficulty in educating children can be seen in

B pre 17: *"I just wanted to find out how to do it right, to try to educate better. Talking is easy, it's doing it that's difficult, I don't know what to do anymore, what am I going to do? It's very difficult to educate.*

Her expression reveals her own individual vulnerability when it comes to being an adequate educator as a mother. I understand her restlessness to find a better way of educating. It reveals the dichotomy between the theory of educating and the difficult practice of practicing it, which translates into constant uncertainty.

It is worth highlighting Zagury (2001, p. 31), when he emphasizes that educating involves a new challenge every day. Bringing up a child is a very complex process, with unexpected situations for most parents, who never dreamed of having so much work to do, every day, every hour of the day.

1.4 Subcategory the way of educating Correlated with the child's level of development

The idea expressed by subject D pre 5 reveals that it is difficult to educate children due to their lack of critical reflexive thinking, as is expected of adults. *"Children don't really think properly. They think. But not like adults. They don't think like us, so it's difficult to educate them."*

This statement refers to the mother's lack of knowledge about the peculiarities of the child's growth and development, as she compares the child's thinking to that of an adult and demonstrates a sense of devaluation regarding the child's thinking. The mother reduces the child in an attempt to express that the adult's thinking is adequate and the child's is not.

I understand that, during childhood, children go through different stages of growth and development, acquiring and perfecting skills to understand the world around them. However, the caregiver responsible in this study, the mothers, often find it difficult to understand the particularities of this child, to perceive him or her as a distinct person who discovers the world and builds his or her own knowledge in a gradual and growing evolutionary process. My professional practice allows me to state that, most of the time, a child is punished for behaviour that is perfectly appropriate and desirable for their stage of development, but which, however, is not recognized as appropriate by the adult carers, because they lack knowledge about the child's stage of personality development.

Amen (2005, p.45) points out that, contrary to what many people believe, children are not born as "blank pages", bringing their own personalities and characteristics into the family relationship, because a child is born with their own temperament, sleep and vigilance cycle, level of tolerance, sensitivity to touch and noise, resistance to infections, abilities to adapt to change, and need for affection. Similarly, parents enter the relationship with their child bringing their own temperaments, sleep and vigilance cycle, level of tolerance, sensitivity to touch and noise, resistance to infections, abilities to adapt to change, need for affection, previous experiences with other children.

According to Thompson and Ashwill (1996, p. 16), a child's development refers to an increase in the complexity of forms or functions, and the family greatly influences their physical and emotional development. The development of each child's personality must be known to the adult, as this is fundamental to their education. When the use of discipline is based on the child's individual qualities, it is more likely to be effective; however, I can see from the statements obtained in the interviews that parents lack knowledge about their children's personality development, including how the child's personality can also affect their interaction with their parents. This was evident in the testimony of subject B pre 3: *"Punishment is good because it makes the child think, depending on their age. From 1 to 10 years old, they don't understand much, they understand more with a spanking. You're not going to punish a two-year-old, they won't understand. Besides, that kid is terrible, he won't sit still and that annoys me too much*". However, this same mother, at another point in the interview, subject B pre 44, emphasized her difficulty in educating her son and related the act of hitting to physical aggression, in line with the TV campaign against child violence, *"I can't give him punishment, he won't understand. If I hit him, he'll get worse. How am I going to educate him? It's on TV every day, that's violence against children.*

It's worth remembering what Muszkat (2002, p. 172) warns us about public policies aimed at children and adolescents, which exclude their main nucleus of insertion: the family,

Category: Forms of Education in Practice

In this second category of the first dimension of the study, we find the interviewees' answers to the question about the forms of education they knew and used with their children in practice, divided into four subcategories: from dialog to shouting; intimidation to corporal punishment; physical aspects; and psychological aspects, as shown in Chart 2,

Table 2- **Forms of Education in Practice**

Category	Subcategory
2 Forms of Education in Practice	2.1 from dialogue to shouting 2.2 intimidation for corporal punishment 2.3 physical aspects 2.4 psychological aspects

Source: Interviews with the responsible aggressors before taking part in the workshops (2005),

2.1 Subcategory from dialogue to shouting

Subjects A pre 33 and B pre 71 have an intrinsic harshness in their communication with their children, evidenced by the commonplace act of shouting.

Subject A pre 33 said: *"Instead of talking to my children, I shout. My mother says I shout too much at the children. I know that, but I don't know how to do it differently".*

Subject B pre 71 said: *"I get annoyed with my little one and shout: Shut up! I'd like to talk, but I can't, I just shout at him".*

The analysis of these two testimonies shows that the mothers are aware that they yell at their children too much and that they would like to stop doing it; however, in practice, they don't succeed.

I understand that verbal aggression is a specific form of violence against children and stands out for its incidence, pertinence and action, reducing the child's psychosocial functioning.

Vissing (1991) defines verbal aggression as communication intended to cause psychological pain to another person or communication perceived as having this intention. In this sense, it considers two subtypes of verbal aggression. Instrumental verbal aggression, in which the aggressor aims to put an end to undesirable conduct by uttering pejorative words or symbols that are dissonant with proper communication (e.g. Shut up, you donkey), and expressive verbal aggression, in which the aggressor uses pejorative expressions with the sole aim of denigrating the child (e.g. You're no good).

According to the Ministry of Health (2002, p.20), psychological violence includes any action or omission that causes damage to a person's self-esteem, identity or development.

Psychological violence, in this study, is the hierarchical relationship that subjects the child to the power of the adult, demonstrated by shouting and punishment, because this is when the adult decides and imposes their interests, expectations and feelings. Thus, in this area of violence, a relationship of domination is established which has a disciplinary character, in other words, there is a desire on the part of the adult to teach the child socially accepted norms and behaviors.

Interpersonal relationships in the child's socialization process become violent when the adult's use of power is exacerbated.

I believe that psychological violence is one of the most common forms of violence practiced against children and perhaps one of the most difficult to recognize, due to its subjective nature and the fact that it doesn't present visible marks that are easy to observe, as is the case with physical violence.

Manifested in different ways, it is present in all situations of violence, causing adverse effects on the child's physical and psychosocial development, as well as on the stability of their personality, with a consequent decrease in self-esteem.

Briggs (2002, p.5) defines self-esteem as the way a person feels about themselves; it is the general judgment they make of themselves, how much they like themselves. The author refers to the importance of self-esteem in a child's life, because self-esteem "is the spring that propels the child towards success or failure as a human being."

2.2 Subcategory for corporal punishment

Subject B pre 43 said: *"With my little son I cursed all the time, I used to take the quince stick, but I didn't hit him, I always just threatened him, just showed him".*

From the above account, I can see the mother's behavior of frightening and repressing, associated with the possibility of hitting the child. This exemplifies the idea of the power that adults exercise over children. It also demonstrates the frequency and banality with which this type of violence occurs. The act of cursing and intimidating a child justifies action that does not focus on aspects relating to child protection measures and integrity. In the same vein, subject E pre 50 said: *"I count to two with my girls and they usually obey, because they know that if I count to three they'll get beaten".*

I notice, in both the statements expressed in this subcategory, the mothers' difficulties in setting limits, "which means defining rules or guidelines for behavior" (Whaley and Wong, 1989, p.259).

Instead of proposing positive and interactive components, mothers present their threats in a negative way, introducing fear and the automatization of behaviors they have established into the family relationship. In this way, the mother is not there to protect them from possible problems with their impulses for freedom, but to prevent them from experiencing their own situations and exploring their world.

I think that the practice of humiliating a child, of making them undeserving of affection, respect and protection, on the part of the adult, indicates the urgent need to provide adequate means and strategies to intervene as early as possible in these cases and prevent the appearance of other associated forms of violence.

I believe that every child is a physically fragile human being, incapable of protecting themselves and dependent on adults to reveal their potential, and that this can only be done properly if their biological and psychological needs are met.

Children are born helpless and depend on their parents for their survival for a long time, so they will have to go through many stages to complete their development. For development to take place in a healthy way, the child needs a family environment that encourages it.

An adequate relationship between the child and their parents is seen as a necessary condition for the child's satisfactory development of feelings such as trust and self-control, problem-solving skills, as well as maintaining and establishing future relationships.

It is important to emphasize the role that parents play as role models for this child;

their influence, whether beneficial or not, in childhood will generally have repercussions throughout life.

I understand that the act of an adult swearing at a child, intimidating them and physically punishing them shows that adults are unaware of how this practice can have negative repercussions on the child's emotional development, making them an insecure person in the future.

Corroborating this idea, Santos (1998) points out that psychological violence is the most commonly practiced form of violence and can cause serious damage to the child's emotional and social development.

2.3 Physical aspects subcategory

In this subcategory, the interviewees expressed the use of physical punishment as a way of preventing certain behavior by the child. It should be noted that this subcategory comprises the largest number of statements represented in the study, due to the large number of times it was mentioned. Therefore, the excerpts from the interviews will be presented in the order in which they were highlighted, separated in sequence by the five subjects interviewed.

Subject A mentioned the use of physical force against children on five separate occasions during the interview (Subject A pre 27, A pre 32, A pre 40, A pre 49, A pre 44), noting that both she and her mother (maternal grandmother) hit the children, but the locations differed. While the grandmother spanks the buttocks, the mother spanks in general. I also noticed that the age of the child was not a factor that prevented them from hitting their children. *"They are beaten because there is no other way". "When my mother hits my girls it's only on the buttocks, not me. I take them by the arm, shake them and hit them on the legs, the ass, everything. "They scream more than I hit them". "I counted two spankings I gave my baby". "I just go and slap them so they obey me".*

In Subject B's accounts, I noticed that she used physical force against the children six different times during the interview; she alternated between the places where she hit and the means used to hit. Although she reports that it is for educational purposes, she also mentions the anger that moved her to the act of hitting. (Subject B; pre 5, B pre 11, B pre 22, B pre 61, B pre 66 and B pre 68) *"I hit his little hands. Then I explain to him that he's been beaten up so he won't do it again". "It was straight in the ass, but it was with so much anger that it really hurt." "I always hit him in the ass, I do, so he can learn." "I get him angry, I give him a few jolts and then I hit him." "He's scary, he only needs to be slapped obey. "I have no patience with him, I slap him, I've hit him with a slipper, with a belt."*

Subject C's statements demonstrate the use of physical force against children, revealed three different times during the interview (Subject C pre 3, C pre 10, C pre 22), which, as well as being inappropriate, like the other subjects, is accompanied by uncontrolled impulses that have resulted in exacerbations and complications, going as far as beating: *"The last time was with a stick. I've beaten my daughter". "Sometimes I hit her with my hand, sometimes with a slipper, sometimes with a belt." "I've beaten her a lot, twice. The last time she almost died if it hadn't been for her aunt helping.*

Subject D's speech revealed similar aspects to those expressed by the other mothers; however, she emphasized that she was influenced by the punitive culture of spanking as an educational practice in the context where she lives. The use of physical force against children was mentioned five times during the interview (Subject D pre 3, D pre 6, D pre 1 3, D pre 14, D pre 17). It was clear that there are pre-established conditions for hitting the child in the mouth and the practice of justifying to the child the punishment they will suffer. *"Before you hit, you have to explain to the child why you are hitting. The child has to know why they are being hit." "As soon as you say a word, you get a slap on the mouth, if you disobey, you get a slap". "At least where I live, that's the way it is, people educate by hitting their children, we spank them, we take the slipper when we need it." "Sometimes I hit and it hurts, not to the point of breaking an arm, but it hurts, to the point of turning purple, you can see the marks, even on my hand." "You start by hitting them in the mouth and it goes from there, it's more like physical aggression, you give them a few shakes, a few slaps, you start beating them when you lose control.*

Subject E reported using physical force against children on four separate occasions during the interview (Subject E pre 28, E pre 33, E pre 45, E pre 59): *"I end up saying things I shouldn't say and hitting them". 'ever since I was a little girl, I used to hit them a few months ago". "I explain first, if I have to say it again I go and hit them". "Sometimes I hit both my daughters and only one had to be hit. "I've hit them with my hand, with my slipper, with a belt and a buckle"*. Her testimonies also reveal that sometimes physical aggression goes hand in hand with verbal inappropriateness. She also recognizes that the physical punishment that she considers deserved at the moment only for one daughter is extended to her sister as well.

The act of hitting the child was reported by all five interviewees. This behavior used by the children's parents is based on physical superiority, on the power they have over the child, and conveys the idea that aggression against children is a valid way to resolve a given situation.

I believe that when an adult hits a child, regardless of the area of the child's body that is hit, regardless of the force applied, using their hand or any other instrument, what is actually happening is abuse, the use of physical force to dominate a child. It should also be noted that this method has the limitation that children grow up all the time and parents don't; therefore, in order to maintain some advantage, parents will need to use increasingly elaborate accessories to achieve some effect; in other words, violence follows a progressive and ascending scale. The mother may start with a spanking to stop some behavior and, after a few days, she will be using the slipper to stop the same behavior.

Zagury (2002, p.127) warns us that the tendency of parents is to start hitting more, trying to achieve the effect initially achieved with a spanking. This idea is in line with what Deslandes (1994) proposes about physical violence, which is characterized by any single or repeated action, not accidental (or intentional), perpetrated by an adult or older aggressor, which causes physical harm to a child or adolescent. This harm, caused by the abusive act, can range from mild injury to extreme consequences, such as death.

Consulting the existing literature on physical violence, especially in the last twenty years, I note that the concept that most authors have emphasized is that physical violence is any action that causes physical pain to a child, from shaking, slapping to a fatal beating.

The discussion on the nature of the conceptual issue of physical violence is of fundamental importance in this research, since I understand that any manifestation of the use of physical force by an adult to intentionally cause some kind of pain to a child constitutes violence.

I believe that the use of physical violence against children is part of the idea that violence consists of an unequal interrelationship of forces; it is a form of domination exercised against them, which reduces their condition to that of an object, thus denying their condition as a full subject of rights.

I emphasize that an adult will always have other disciplinary options than using physical force against the child.

It is necessary to emphasize, then, that among the forms of physical violence used, which range from spanking to beating, I perceive the manifestation of a practice that is cultural and still accepted by segments of society, thus being used as an educational and disciplinary method.

The national TV program Fantastico, aired on October 9, 2000, showed a poll that revealed the acceptance of the practice of parents hitting their children as a form of education. The data linked to this information network showed that the act of spanking was accepted by 61% of the parents who took part in the spontaneous popular poll. (Source: Rede Globo de Televisão).

The violence that parents practice against their children has been reproduced throughout the history of civilization and has consolidated a culture that incorporates the act of hitting children as something natural.

The quote by Gomes and Filho (2004 p. 17) is a warning when they point out that violence is perpetuated in families, especially against children, where instead of being recognized as something to be combated, it is considered a manifestation of care, love and an instrument of education.

2.4 Psychological aspects subcategory

Encouraging detachment from the father figure, used as a way of easing the situation of inattention in order to visit the daughters, makes the mother take ownership of the psychological violence, as can be seen in the testimony of subject E pre 69: *"I say to my daughter: Forget it, forget your father. Pretend he's dead. He doesn't give you a lift anymore, he likes you better, forget about him. His delay in visiting the girls annoys me".*

This testimony emphasizes how children are treated within the family and how violent the relationship between family members is.

The mother has difficulties in dealing with the child's requests regarding the delay in the presence of the father, who is in semi-open prison, so she expresses her feelings of frustration in an inappropriate way, acting out of control on impulse.

In this mother's account, we can clearly see the social situation of family vulnerability experienced by this family. The use of speech with a symbolic connotation of violence may correspond, in this context, to a resource widely used by society, since it is a type of behavior that manifests itself as a way of communicating for many people. It is often the only form of language that exists in the relationship dynamics of many families. Most of the time, I believe that no parent wants their child to suffer; they just end up acting as they can and, on many occasions, this represents the use of some kind of violence, actually demonstrating a kind of weakness, rather than strength. Intra-family relationships are the deepest and most significant thing that exists for human beings; in line with Elsen (1999), I can say that in families where there is some form of violence against children, the performance of social roles is unstable.

In another excerpt from the interview with this same subject, which deserves to be highlighted for the psychological aspects mentioned, this mother said: *"There was a time when I was thinking of giving up my daughters. Because I couldn't bear to see the children in need any longer. I said to myself, I'm going to give these children to someone who is better able to look after them than I am. When they cried, fought, bothered me, I told them both that I was going to give them away".* Subject E pre 75.

The revelation of the purpose of giving the children up for adoption was linked to moments when the children fought with each other, thus showing adoption as an act of punishment, rather than protection and care.

The way a child is treated within his or her own family can mean that the family is a place where violence, neglect and lack of protection can occur.

In this case, it is contrary to the ECA, in its article 43, when it states that "adoption will be granted when it presents real advantages for the adoptee and is based on legitimate reasons."

I believe that problems such as precarious socio-economic conditions, poor schooling, drug use, the presence of some kind of illness in one of the family members and the excessive stress of modern life are often factors associated with different types of violence against children.

The World Report on Violence and Health (2002, p.80) points out that there is a need for a better understanding of how broader social, cultural and economic factors influence family life. I believe that these forces interact with individual and family factors to produce coercive and violent patterns of behavior. Most of them, however, have been largely neglected in studies on child maltreatment.

Category Motives triggering the violent act

Chart 3 shows the category that deals with the reasons for the violent act and the related subcategories: the psychosocial characteristics of the child; psychosocial characteristics of the adult; fighting between siblings; maintaining power/authority; family dynamics.

Chart 3- Reasons for the violent act

Category	Sub-category
3 Motives that trigger violence	3.1 Psychosocial characteristics of children
	3.2 Adult psychosocial characteristics
	3.3 Brothers fighting
	3.4 Maintaining power/authority
	3.5 Family dynamics

Source: Interviews with perpetrators before taking part in the workshops (2005).

3.1 Subcategory Psychosocial characteristics of the child

The category Children's psychosocial characteristics emerged as reasons for triggering violence, as can be seen below.

Subject A pre 22 said: *"He has a way about him. He's very angry, agitated, irritable". "He's terrible, he'll only obey if he's beaten".* (Subject A pre 24.)

The adult's justification for using any kind of violence against the child was evidenced in the testimonies by the transfer of responsibility for the violent act from the adult to the child.

At various points in the interviews, I observed that the adults blamed themselves for the act they had provoked and linked the cause of their violent behavior to the child's characteristics or to some action the child had taken that required them to react in a disciplinary way.

Subject C pre 4 said: *"When they disobey older people, say bad names, talk back, intrude on adult conversations, say things they don't know". "The children cry, they stress me out, they're always around me reigning over me, kind of getting on my nerves:* (Subject E pre 27.)

I think that adults' explanations of the violence they use against children are an approach specifically related to the question of the trivialization of violence in most cultures.

I agree with Amen (2005), because I believe that violence against children is always a tragedy and can get worse, however, when people ignore the underlying problems that are contributing to the difficulties, to the increase in violence against the child, in other words, interfering in the adjustment of the relationship between parents and children. Therefore, the fact that social influences occur early in a child's life often suggests that special attention should be focused on the process of their development.

I believe that the strategy used by parents to educate a child should always be based on an understanding of the child's motivations for action, of what, at each stage of child development, the child is capable of knowing, what is relevant to feel.

There is a social tolerance expressed by the family's agreement with corporal discipline, since the impression we get from the analysis of the interviews is that the adults don't consider that hitting their children could mean violence; on the contrary, hitting is a trivialized and unappreciated strategy.

In the family contexts analyzed, it was possible to observe aspects that significantly affected the adults so that they used physical force against the child. This situation is made clear in the words of a mother: *"in the case of hitting me, being rude to me, being mean to me, that's wrong, I don't like it". (*Subject B pre 18.)

Subject E pre 20's statement reads: *"eia starts to tease me and won't stop asking me about her father, who is in prison, and the fact that eia is crying because of deie makes me angry, I just have to slap eia to stop, I want to beat the girl to death".*

From the analysis of the interviews, I can see that the use of corporal punishment was a common disciplinary practice. Its application ranged from spanking to beating with a whip.

The "REPORT FOR THE END OF PHYSICAL PUNISHMENTS AGAINST CHILDREN", published in 1996 by the Citizenship and Human Rights Commission of the Legislative Assembly of the State of Rio Grande do Sul, brings up an important question proposed by Soder, member and president of RADDA BARNEN, which is a grassroots movement with more than 80,000 people across Sweden, founded in 1919, independent of ideologies, political parties and religions, funded by public contributions to safeguard its independence from government authorities. It works for children in Sweden and the developing world, involving children living in particularly difficult circumstances.

The programs benefit street children, refugees and children in armed conflicts, supporting the care of mothers and children. It fights racism and all forms of violence, defending children's rights until they reach the age of 18.

Regarding the reasons why so many parents still beat their children, Soder (1996) states that it is because these parents are showing their children the stresses that emanate from adult societies that are far from being family-friendly and, in part, because they cannot think of any other way of disciplining their children.

It should be mentioned that there has been an increase in the application of different corporal punishments in various cultures throughout the history of civilization.

Kadushin and Martin (1981), in a study carried out in the United States, cited in the report in question (1996, p.84), concluded that all physical abuse of children begins with a slap, a push from the father or mother, which doesn't mean "abuse", but which escalates when the child doesn't respond to the parents' wishes.

3.2 Subcategory adult psychosocial characteristics sources of tension

The psychosocial characteristics of the perpetrator, as reported in the interviews, are those which generate tension and stress, such as impatience, uncontrolled impulses, irritability and a feeling of helplessness in the maternal role. *"I work all day, I get home late and I'm stressed, they want attention, they won't sit still, they won't cooperate with you, I can't control myself and I hit them".* (Subject A pre 38.)

"I'm very nervous, I lash out. I have no patience with children. I get angry easily, sometimes even with the tone of my voice, if the toy is agitated it bothers me." (Subject B pre 13.)

"I was nervous about other things that had happened, and at the end of the stress, I picked her up and hit her a lot, I ended up taking it out on her," (Subject C pre21).

"I have panic, we suffer prejudice with this mental illness, so educating the girls is more difficult with my problem". (Subject E pre 83.)

Amen (2005) points out that parents are subjected to stress linked to marital relationships, health, work, finances, transportation, among others. Therefore, this author believes that the complexities of education involve the characteristics of the child associated with the characteristics of the parents, added to the social stresses, resulting in the combination of the relationship between parents and children.

I believe that the child has a series of demands, such as food, a lap, attention, and that they depend exclusively on their parents or someone who replaces them to meet their needs in order for them to grow and develop properly, aspects that are not consistent with the family dynamics of the interviewees.

The possibility of intervening in the phenomenon of intrafamily violence represents a fundamental moment in the life of any family, since I believe that the practice of violence is associated with different factors.

Given the complexity of the problem, it is essential that professionals focus their attention on the indicators that trigger intrafamily violence, requiring a specific response to the needs highlighted.

Magalhães (2004) points to risk factors for violence against children which can act as unspecific indicators and which are often associated, increasing the risk of intrafamily violence. In this context, she indicates individual characteristics of the parents, also found in our study, such as an abusive pattern of alcohol and other drugs, immature and impulsive personality, low self-control and reduced tolerance of frustration, as well as great vulnerability to stress, intolerant attitudes, [...] Cp.45).

Barudy (1997) reports that parents who do not take adequate care of their children show significant deficiencies in their parental functions, which can be the result of three dynamics that are mixed together: biological, cultural and contextual, circumstances that are also similar to those experienced by the subjects of this study.

The World Report on Violence and Health (2002) points out that research has linked child violence to certain characteristics of the person responsible for the child, as well as characteristics of the family environment. While some factors, including demographic characteristics, are related to variations in risk, others are related to the psychological and behavioral characteristics of the person caring for the child or to aspects of the family environment that can compromise parenthood and lead to child abuse.

3.3 Subcategory Fighting between brothers

The frequent fights between the siblings were mentioned by those responsible as one of the triggers for them to intervene. The problem lies in the way they intervened.

"They grab each other and fight over everything. I try to separate them and I can't, I just have to hit them to stop them fighting." (Subject A pre 16-)

*"She's terrible, she hit her little sister with her sandal, hitting her little sister is what she does the most." (*Subject A pre 50.)

"They fight a lot. They fight over toys, they fight over everything, they even fight for no reason". (Subject E pre 86.)

I think it's the parents' job to prevent children from hurting each other; however, how these parents act will depend on whether the situation normalizes or deteriorates.

Many parents are frightened by their children's aggression, fearing that this behavior is a harbinger of violent and antisocial behavior in the future. However, in order to deal with this behavior, it is essential to understand the reasons for the child's aggression. Sometimes children repeat acts that they observe in adults, i.e. children from violent homes tend to use aggression as a means of getting what they want, or as a reaction to a tense situation.

In this sense, Amen (2005) points out that children who have been verbally, physically, emotionally or sexually abused lose their emotional bonds and their sense of limits, and are therefore more likely to lash out when frustrated, because that's what others have done to them.

Fights between siblings are ways of seeking power, autonomy, importance and individuality

I believe it's the parents' job to recognize that each child has his or her own identity and therefore they should treat each child differently, never comparing one child to another.

Tiba (2002) points out that trying to find out who is responsible for the fight in order to punish them is usually impossible, as everyone has reasonable arguments that they are victims and it is always the other person's fault. He points out that punishments don't solve fights between siblings, but taking responsibility for the consequences and compensating for the damage caused can educate a lot.

According to Zagury (2002), parents ask themselves in anguish why there is verbal or physical aggression between their children, they feel a kind of moral pain when they see their children fighting, it's as if they haven't managed to convey the notion of family to them.

3.4 Subcategory maintaining power/authority

I see difficulties in the family relationships these guardians have with their children. The impression one gets from analyzing the testimonies is that they know they have to set limits for their children, but they have problems with how to set these limits correctly, not least because they associate children's obedience with the use of physical force.

"I keep telling her not to do it, but the child continues. First I ground her, but it's no use, the bad behavior continues, she fights me, retorts. Then I go and hit her to put an end to the problem. (Subject A pre 4 1.)

"I have to put an end to the situation. I'm the adult. I'm the mother, I'm the one who knows things". (Subject A pre I 2.)

"I tell him he can't go out. It's the same as nothing. He goes, he's cheeky, I run after him, I tell him he can't do it like that and I give him a spanking to show him that I'm in charge and he has to obey'. (Subject B pre 65.)

"When we're very aggressive, angry, they become aggressive too. They raise their hands to hit you, you can't let them. You're the mother, you have to hit them, not them you." (Subject C pre 5.)

I believe that anyone responsible for a child, whether a parent, wants to be able to pass on their values and standards to their children, so that they grow and develop satisfactorily, becoming suitable and happy adults in the future. For this to happen, parents need to exercise their parental authority, setting clear limits with the child in order to achieve their educational goals.

It is necessary to bring up the idea of Zagury (2002), when she warns that, when talking about limits, many people interpret this as a license to exercise an authoritarian stance, total control or even violence. The author emphasizes the difficulty in knowing when authority ends and authoritarianism begins; however, she explains that an authoritarian is someone who exercises power using only their point of view, physical strength or the power that gives them their position.

Omer (2002, p. 13) defines parental authority as the parents' ability to establish rules and values for the child and to prevent acts that might subvert them. Thus, explains the author, any type of parent, modern or old-fashioned, lay or religious, aspires to authority and may prefer to support it in blind obedience or rational discussion, in rewarding or punishing behavior, in setting a positive or negative example; however, without authority, parents cannot transmit their standards to their children.

3.5 Family dynamics subcategory

Social exclusion, combined with withdrawal from social life, conflicts and family helplessness, have generated life circumstances with suffering that are conducive to physical violence.

"My mother was ill, I was alone, I isolated myself from everyone, I ended up taking my problems out on the children". (Subject A pre 9.)

"I have to study, work, I don't have anyone to help me with my children." (Subject C pre 77.)

"Everything is difficult for me, we sleep badly on very thin mattresses, the floor is damp, there are lots of mosquitoes down there, it seems to be getting worse and

worse, the circle is closing more and more. I depend on my mother for everything, I hear abuse from her, from my brother, I've already been beaten by him, I have to put up with everything with my head down because of my daughters". (Subject E pre 38.)

"There were times when I thought about killing myself, I cried day and night, I didn't want to live anymore. I wondered why God wanted me in the world, I'm no use for anything, I'm like an amoeba, I can't even work". (Subject E pre 78.)

I realize that the family with violence in its internal dynamics must be understood within a context that involves a complexity of cultural, social and economic determinants.

The interviews show that the economic, social and structural difficulties experienced by these mothers affect the children differently through their impact on parental behavior and the availability of family resources.

Magalhàes (2004) mentions the characteristics of the family context that generate sources of tension, such as single-parent families, reconstituted families, unstructured families with dysfunctional relationships between the parents, crises in family life and families with socio-economic problems and no support in the extended family.

By analyzing these four statements, it is possible to see the economic oppression that means that today, despite the great technical and scientific development, significant portions of our society are marked by suffering that establishes violence as a constant in individual and social relationships, since there is an evident loss of material quality of life, deprivation determined by the high unemployment rate, great concentration of income and cultural impositions determining the relationship between individuals.

Therefore, I believe, like Rosàrio (1999), that contemporary society exposes human beings to situations of violence and high social risk, since the process that produces the framework of economic exclusion sustains, at the same time, the diminishing role of the state, minimizing its public functions and transforming it into a body subordinate to the interests of large transnational economic corporations, emphasizing that the difficulties experienced by these families are linked to the greater violence that dominates them.

In this way, I can see that Brazilian society is organized and determined by an exclusionary capitalist economic model, characterized by a high concentration of income, which is one of the main factors of inequality that generate differences, causing privileges and, consequently, the absence of fundamental rights for many.

According to the World Report on Violence and Health (2002, p. 671), parents who commit physical abuse are more likely to be young, single, poor, unemployed and have a lower level of education than their partners. In both developed and industrialized countries, poor and young single mothers are among those most at risk of using violence against their children.

Category: Family History

Chart 4 shows the category dealing with family history and the subcategories related to it: past/current family history; family intervention in the face of violence; awakening to the option of professional help.

Chart 4- Family history

Category	Subcategory
4 Family history	4.1 Past/current family history
	4.2 Family intervention in the face of violence
	4.3 Awakening to the option of professional help

Source: Interviews with perpetrators before taking part in the workshops (2005).

4.1 Subcategory past/current family history

From analyzing the testimonies, I can see that the mothers who used physical violence against their children had a history of child abuse. The phenomenon of multigenerationality occurred, i.e. the phenomenon whereby the child who was exposed to violence, intentionally and repeatedly, became an adult who subjected the children to the same experiences they suffered.

"My father beat me and my brother a lot with punches, kicks and hair-pulling. He beat my mother too. (Subject A pre 1.)

"My God, if I did that to my mother, she'd slap me across the face". (Subject A pre 3 1.)

"My father was violent, I was about five years old and I asked him for a pencil to draw with, he turned around and kicked me and I flew into the wall, I remember it to this day". Subject B pre 27.

"My mother used to beat me with a stick. There were marks on our bodies, it hurt a lot. She raised me as if I were a child. If she told you to go there, you had to go. If you didn't, the lasso would catch you". (Subject B pre 69 .)

"They beat me all the time. My father beat me a lot. With anything in front of him, a slipper, a belt, a knife sheath. But it was my father, my late mother didn't beat me much". (Subject C pre 15.)

"I didn't really speak a word, but all the other wrong things I did, I was always beaten up. I was beaten by my mother and my sister. It wasn't just a slap, I was even beaten on the legs with a sledgehammer". (Subject D pre 9.)

*"I was never beaten by my father. The little education I have is because I was beaten by my mother, I used to go to school with purple legs." (*Subject E pre 5 1.)

Caminha (1999) points out that multigenerationality is a variable that deserves to be highlighted in the issue of violence, given its recurrence, since adults with traumatic experiences carry a cognitive and behavioral pattern learned in their childhoods, of inadequate functioning with the children they live with. Thus, the child uses the adult's referential model to behave and form representations and affections, not least because the first years of life are only experienced with a referential family nucleus, so there are no other comparative behavioral parameters. The author also states that it would be correct to say that children and adolescents exposed to intentional and repetitive violence learn these patterns as truths, and these internal truths, affective representational mental patterns, will be the mediators of their social relationships; this is the origin of the phenomenon of multigenerationality. (p.46)

According to the international literature, represented by Furniss (1993), Green (1995) and Flores (1998), when there is the phenomenon of multigenerationality, it happens that these adults, when relating to children, tend to be negligent or abusive as well.

Caminha (1999, p. 57) expands on this, saying that in female behavior there is a strong tendency to form emotional bonds with people who have the same personality profile as the aggressor, demonstrating that the models formed in childhood are very strong. For this author, female behavior shows a strong tendency towards depression, suicide, alcoholism and drug addiction. In cases of sexual abuse, prostitution is significant. With regard to male behavior, there is a strong tendency towards offending behavior, especially in adolescents and young adults, a time when alcohol and drug abuse is very high. He also describes that, in samples involving women admitted to psychiatric hospitals, the patients (between 22% and 57%) had been victims of abuse in childhood.

In this way, I can say that the childhood family histories of the subjects of the study were shaped by the practice of domestic violence and were the precursors to their current aggressive actions.

4.2 Subcategory Family intervention in the face of violence

This subcategory, which refers to family influences interfering in the interruption of violence, becomes a paradox in relation to the previous subcategory, when the family of origin refers to attitudes of physical aggression.

From the testimony of the mothers who used violence against their children, I can see the need for advice and intervention from their close family members in terms of encouragement and restrictions to stop this practice.

*"My mother always tells me that I won't be able to raise my children properly, that you can't achieve things by hitting them all the time. But that's just the way I am. (*Subject B prè 54.)

"When I was married, I had never spanked the children. My ex-husband wouldn't even allow me to spank them. He defended the girls" (Subject C prè 12.)

"I started taking medication. My mother insisted, so I started to get better, to control myself more". (Subject E prè 10.)

The approach to the family, such as the mother (grandmother) and the ex-husband, has been a necessary form of intervention, based on delimiting criteria that refer to both the educational consequences for the child and the frequency and intensity of the aggression.

The fact that the family is a space for coexistence doesn't mean that, in many cases, it has a democratic style for resolving conflictive situations and therefore resorts to its personal collection of procedures acquired in the learning process itself. However, family life can be very valuable, especially in times of crisis.

Tiba (2002) states that grandparents play a complementary role in the education of parents, a fact that is demonstrated in our families.

I believe that different characteristics of adult personality and behavior have been associated with violence against children. These characteristics compromise the exercise of motherhood and are associated with the breakdown of marital, parental and social relationships, the lack of ability to deal with the stressors of everyday life and the difficulty in obtaining support from other family members and the community.

Parents' capacity for education and family life is very vulnerable to daily stress.

Amen (2005) points out that pressure at work, financial problems, discord between the couple or health problems can interfere with the ability to raise children.

One subject in the study needed maternal insistence to adhere to specialized treatment, in this case medication. Prado and colleagues describe the successful experience of drug intervention for impulse control in cases of abusive mothers.

The World Report on Violence and Health (2002) points out that parents who are more likely to physically abuse their children tend to have low self-esteem, poor impulse control, mental health problems and anti-social behavior.

For Whaley and Wong (1989), in order for the family to be able to cope with tensions and problems, each of its members must receive support so that each part of the family system is strengthened. He goes on to say that the family's greatest strength lies in the support that each of its members provides to each other.

4.3 Subcategory awakening to the option of professional help

There are many reasons why people go to a health service; however, in these two testimonies, the reasons are fundamentally linked to the conditions of these women, who are helpless in relation to the exercise of motherhood.

"You can see how far I've come. I was angry with my son. I didn't know what to do with my life. I felt very alone. By the time I got help, it was too late. I don't think it could have gotten that bad. It was only here in hospital that I found help". (Subject B pre 32.)

I came to ask for help because I was at the end of my tether. I almost killed my daughter and all I could think about was killing myself too". (Subject C pre 27.)

Both used physical violence to discipline the children and, when confronted, explained to the health team that they used physical violence as a way of curbing the children's bad behavior.

These mothers felt unprepared for the maternal role and showed a lot of impotence, lack of control and irritation in response to their children's behavior.

Elsen (2004) points out that when we think about violence against children, violence in the family, we have to work on some myths. One of them is the myth of maternal love, which doesn't accept that there are mothers who find it difficult to accept their child, that it's not every mother who loves, that it's not every child who is loved by their mother. We need to review the maternal instinct, recognizing that it is not innate.

Another issue that the author addresses as a myth is the fact that we think parents always know what's best for their children, as if they were born knowing how to look after, love and educate them.

Varela (2004) points out that, in situations of violence, the success of any conventional situation will depend on what it means to live in a family and in society, to be born, to live and to develop in this world, on the meaning that life has for these people and on the skills they have acquired to get on in life and in the reality in which life is concretely expressed,

The World Report on Violence and Health (2002) reports that stress resulting from job changes, loss of income, health problems or other aspects of the family environment can increase the level of conflict in the home and the ability to deal with these conflicts or find support, which is the reality of the interviewees.

I realize that intrafamily violence against children is a serious health problem, which makes the hospital a point of reference in dealing with the problem, because I agree with Farinati (1993) when he points out that the hospital is a privileged place for observation, protection, confirmation or information of presumptions that allows decisions to be made about the family crisis, as well as obviously offering specialized treatment.

In situations involving intrafamily violence, I believe it is necessary to train education and health professionals in their ethical, professional and citizenship obligations in dealing with this problem. In this direction, it is important to emphasize the recommendation of the ECA, in its article 245, regarding the obligation of these professionals to report any suspicion or confirmation of ill-treatment of children.

Above all, I believe that health education in the care of families in situations of intrafamily violence should not be restricted only to professionals working in hospitals, but mainly to education and health professionals working in the various potential settings for family encounters, such as schools, health centers and the community.

In this sense, I agree with Waidman, Decesaro and Marcos (2004) when they point out that it is important to discuss the role of the health service in the community, because in some way it interferes in the situation of violence in three ways: in the structuring of services offered to the population, an obligation guaranteed in the Brazilian Federal Constitution; in the ethical issue, as it involves the professional-family-individual relationship; and in the alteration of family dynamics, mobilized by unmet basic needs.

The "Declaration of the Rights of the Child" is based on Article 7, which states that the best interests of the child will be the guiding principle for those responsible for education and guidance; this responsibility lies primarily with the parents.

18. SECOND DIMENSION: POST-WORKSHOPS

In the second dimension of the study, two categories are presented: Experiencing the workshops; and repercussions of the workshops. Both emerged from the testimonies collected after the workshops.

The fifth category of this study deals with participants' experiences of the workshops. From the experiences of these participants, it was possible to obtain two subcategories: the meaning of participation and the acquisition of knowledge, as shown in Chart 5.

Category: Experiencing the Workshops

Chart 5- Experiencing the Workshops

Category	Subcategory
5 Experiencing the workshops	5.1 The meaning of participating in the workshops
	5.2 The acquisition of knowledge

Source: Interviews with the perpetrators after taking part in the workshops (2005).

5.1 Subcategory the meaning of taking part in the workshops

I believe that the interviewees' experience of the workshops was an important one, which brought meaning to reflection and reconstruction in their lives. The analysis of these six fragments of interviews given by each subject shows that they accept the positive meaning of their participation.

"It was great to take part in the workshops. I learned a lot, it helped me a lot, I know that I have good and bad things in me, I still have to improve more, control myself". (Subject A post 1.)

"I've learned a lot of good things, it's important for people's lives." (Subject B post 2)

"I think it's good for us to live better and for our family". (Subject B post 3.)

"I thought it was nice to take part, I really enjoyed it. It's a lot calmer for me now, things are better with myself and the children". (Subject C 1.)

"I learned a lot, it helped me a lot. In the workshops you discover that there are other people with the same problem as you. If they have the same problem as you, you'll see how that person solves it and put it together with the ideas of the professionals who are there to help you, so you start to develop more and improve your problem".

(Subject D post 7.)

There was a resonance in the common reality faced by the participants, in line with the reflections and orientations raised by the professionals.

In this way, the aggressors expressed that they had learned strategies that improved their ability to care for their children.

From the words of these mothers who took part in the workshops because they were in a situation of domestic violence, it can be deduced that a process of reversing these conditions has already begun in their lives, as they say that, with the help they got from the workshops, they improved themselves and their relationships with the children.

One of the objectives of the workshops was to strengthen family ties in order to reduce and/or eradicate the problem of diagnosed intrafamily violence and to provide support for positive changes in family relationships.

Professional interdisciplinarity allowed the convergence of specific perspectives on the needs of the mothers that emerged in the context of the workshops, contributing to the resignification of a new way of interacting with and caring for children.

Among the justifications for interdisciplinarity in health and education is that most health problems require intervention from various perspectives, because the factors that trigger them are diverse and interrelated. It requires an approach from different professionals, allowing for coordination and interaction of all points of view (Gonzales Serrano, 1998).

The professionals who took part in the workshops included a public prosecutor, a doctor, nurses, social workers, psychologists, a recreationalist and trainees in nursing, social work and psychology.

"What everyone in the team told me was very important, it improved my life, I was going through a very difficult time, my husband was in prison, I had no money, no job, I was fighting too much with my mother and brother, I was desperate, I didn't know what to do, I didn't have any patience with my daughters, I was taking everything out on them, my worry, my anger with life". (Subject E 6.)

Through the analysis of these testimonies, I think it's possible to say that the participants perceived and felt themselves to be people who, although they face the reality of intrafamily violence in their daily lives, whether in the role of aggressor or victim, discovered possibilities for alternatives to healthy relationships with their children and family.

The work carried out during the workshops was intended to sensitize and raise awareness among the participants, confronting the reality they had experienced and creating the capacity for new models of social organization in terms of reformulating personal, family and group ties.

The workshops covered discussions of the experiences of violence in their families, trying to discover similarities and differences between the subjects, as well as establishing the meaning and implications of these experiences for life, seeking, through trust between the people in the group and the freedom to talk about the phenomenon of intrafamily violence, another form of family relationship.

For Vieira and Volquind (2002), workshops are an interactive practice, combining individual work and a socialized task, as they guarantee unity between theory and practice. They integrate three basic elements: thinking, feeling and acting.

5.2 Subcategory the acquisition of knowledge

I can see that the workshops held with those responsible for aggression have made it possible to build up knowledge that opens up new perspectives for treating these children and their families, because fundamentally the workshops are a space for expressing and exercising the daily experiences of these individuals.

"I learned about hygiene habits, health, education, drugs, issues related to children, family, getting along with people, and violence". (Subject A post 2.)

"The most important thing I remember is violence, how we do the wrong thing with children and after we hit them they learn that and they'll hit and fight too, they'll want to solve everything by beating, by force". (Subject B post 4.)

"We talked about how to bring up our children, we talked about the serious problems in our lives". (Subject C post 8.)

"All the subjects discussed were important to me, but I most enjoyed learning how it's best to treat children instead of beating them, educating them properly, we really

*don't know what it's like, nobody teaches us, that's why I enjoyed the workshops, I was able to learn things properly." (*Subject D post 3.)

"We talked about violence in the world, people's rights, what rights each Brazilian has that aren't respected, our difficulties in life, the problems we have with our children, the best way to educate". (Subject E post 2.)

I think that holding the workshops with the perpetrators has enabled them to build up knowledge that opens up new perspectives for dealing with these children and their families, as well as their own existential problems. Fundamentally, the workshops are a space for expressing and exercising the experiences shared in the daily lives of these individuals.

The workshop is a working method that developed teaching-learning actions through interactive processes, creating greater socialization, in which each participant shared their experience with the group, discussing and reflecting on the reports brought, as well as intervening in order to understand the situation exposed and seek subsidies to act, contributing to changes in the reality experienced.

This idea is strengthened by educators Vieira and Volquind (2002) when they emphasize that workshops promote the construction of knowledge through action, as well as reflection in and on action.

Borges (2001, p.71) points out that teaching is conceived as a form of symbolic interaction, a process in which subjects act according to what knowledge means to them. As a result, in order to understand the meanings constructed by subjects, it is also necessary to consider the context in which they interact.

The workshops worked on health education as a transformative social practice because, as a collective construction, it is a place of coexistence that encourages and recognizes the individuality of each participant and situates the human reality experienced in each family and in the social environment, always seeking to interfere in this reality of violence in order to transform it.

Category: Workshop repercussions

The sixth category of this study deals with the repercussions of the workshops, from which it was possible to obtain four subcategories: paths to family resilience; family and social coexistence; preventive aspects; and suggestions, as shown in Chart 6.

Table 6. Repercussions of the workshops

Category	Subcategory
6 Repercussions of the workshops	6.1 Pathways to family resilience 6.2 Family and social interaction 6.3 Preventive aspects 6.4 Suggestions

Source: Interviews with perpetrators after taking part in the workshops (2005).

6.1 Subcategory paths to family resilience

At various points in the post-workshop interviews, the impressions and feelings of the participants were expressed in the sense that the participation had allowed transformations to occur in their relationship with their children, including changes in their own behavior.

"At the park I'm learning a different way of conducting myself, today I think I'm a better mother, I'm calmer, more patient with the children's art. I talk to them more, something I didn't do before". (Subject B post 5.)

"I used to be very angry, but I've improved a lot. The way I dealt with the children, I used to hit them a lot, now I know that there are other ways of dealing with them". (Subject C post 7.)

"I arrived at the workshops very stupid, aggressive, but I left the meetings calmer, seeing things differently. I learned that hitting doesn't help and that talking is the best way". (Subject D post 4.)

As can be seen from the reports, the participants used to use physical aggression against the child, but after the workshops, they reported that this attitude was replaced by the strategy of talking instead of hitting. Another aspect that deserves to be highlighted is the participants' self-reflection. As there was a space for families to reflect on their educational practices, I realized that the parents wanted to educate their children correctly; however, they revealed that they didn't know if the way they were acting was right or wrong.

From this perspective, the workshop was an educational and supportive action for rescuing less violent and healthier interpersonal and family relationships. I realize that the workshops have opened up paths to family resilience, since its construct encompasses vulnerability and regenerative power. "It refers to the family's ability to minimize the disruptive impact of the stressful situation through effects that influence the demands and develop the gathering of resources" (ANTONI and KOLLER, 2000, p. 39).

As for the basic elements for family resilience, these authors point to the inclusion of the process of cohesion, "flexibility, open communication, problem solving and firm belief systems, as well as the support of the community in providing [...], social support and the feeling of being connected to a network of relationships [...]". For the researcher, the latter two are consistent with the functions of the workshops held.

I note that the importance of the workshops was basically to reinforce the healthy aspects of families, to put limits on aggressive behavior, to help people improve their self-esteem and to reflect on the social relevance of this.

In this sense, Vieira and Volquid (2002) point out that the workshop is a social group organized for learning, in which interpersonal exchanges, rich in content and experiences, should promote the search for answers to problems.

6.2 Subcategory family and social life

The subjects interviewed after the workshops reported on how the workshops had influenced their family and social life.

"My relationship with my sister has changed a lot since I did the workshops, we're talking about our children's education, only my mother doesn't understand much yet, I think it's because she's older, it's harder to change her mind". (Subject A post 6.)

"You start to have more patience with everyone, even adults, to understand, to respect more". (Subject D post 9.)

I believe that the work carried out in the workshops has influenced the participants to improve their behavior, attitudes and relationships in line with better family coexistence.

In this sense, it is worth remembering what the ECA states in its article 4: "It is the duty of the family, the community, society in general and the public authorities to ensure, with absolute priority, the realization of rights relating to life, health, food, education, sport, leisure, professional training, culture, dignity, respect, freedom and family and community life."

Violence against children, understood from a historical and critical point of view, leads me to point out that this phenomenon is the result of a series of factors, intra and inter family related, cultural, social, economic and psychological. The emotional conditions of the individuals who live with the child, the fact that they are part of a culture that attributes violence a value to be followed, in which the way to overcome conflicts is through the use of different types of violence, leads to the trivialization of this situation.

The workshops sought to break the cycle of violence experienced by these families, making a joint effort to prevent situations of aggression against children from continuing, as well as to prevent new forms of violence.

As a result, the women who took part in the workshops went from being oppressors to being a source of encouragement and help for their families, starting a process of multiplying cognitive, relational and solidarity learning from the work carried out in the workshops.

"I'm trying to help my brother with his drinking and drug problem". (Subject B post 7.)

In the case of the brother of the perpetrator, I can say that subject B was a support and solidarity network, which, according to (ANTOM and KOLLER, 2000) includes relatives [...].

According to Hawley and De Haan (1996), family activities can act as protection by bringing people closer together.

By spreading the knowledge acquired in the workshops to their families, the subjects became multipliers for positive changes in family relationships (ALGERI et al 2002).

Varela (2004) points out that the work proposal for nurses in this situation should be to value the person in all aspects as someone in the process of self-development in the process of becoming, which occurs through stimulated and mediated human interactions.

The important thing is to create spaces and provide experiences so that the person can become aware of themselves as a person and the subject of their decisions.

6.3 Subcategory preventive aspects

"I had already tried to kill myself, but now I don't want to die anymore, I want to take

care of my children, be a good mother." (Subject A post 5.)

From the analysis of this testimony, I can see that the perpetrator recounts a life situation that happened to her, relating the fact that she wanted to live with her parental expectations in relation to her desire to exercise motherhood properly.

I think that, by taking part in the workshops, this guardian recognized her own abusive behaviour, understood how much she needed professional help and proposed specialized treatment, since she was a depressed mother who didn't use medication. This mother didn't only show aggressive behavior towards her children, but also towards herself, as she had a history of suicide attempts. Oski (1992), in his studies on violence in families, states that physical abuse is more common in families whose mother has attempted suicide.

Prado Lima et al. (2001), in a study carried out on the use of medication to reduce abusive maternal behavior, reported that there was a statistically significant reduction; thus, the author points out that pharmaceutical intervention can improve parental behavior and can become an efficient supplement to the psychological and social treatment of child abuse.

"Now I know how not to hit. I punish, I scold a lot, I even shout, but I don't hit like I used to". (Subject B post 6.)

"I used to hit my daughters for anything, I hit them a lot. Today I try to understand what they're feeling, why they're acting the way they are, we talk a lot, we're patient, there's no need to hit ʲ' (Subject C post 4.)

If there is violence of any kind, or if it is triggered by various predisposing factors, the perpetrator always needs a specific approach, because, in most cases, the situation of frustration experienced by the parent or guardian is the frequent reason for aggression, of which the child is the preferred target.

The World Report on Violence and Health (2002) stresses that recognition and awareness, while essential elements for effective prevention, are only parts of the solution. Prevention efforts and policies must focus directly on children, the people responsible for them and the environment in which they live, in order to prevent future abuse and deal effectively with cases of violence that have occurred.

6.4 Subcategory suggestions

"My brother is very angry. In fact, he needed to go to the workshops to learn as well, to improve his life and that of all of us". (Subject B pos 6-)

"There are people who need treatment, who need to be monitored all their lives. I know I'm one of them, I'm sure I've changed, for the better, the important thing is to achieve this with more people in your family, with your neighbors. Everyone should have the opportunity to do the workshops, the children's school teachers, it would be important". (Subject D pos 11.)

From the analysis of these statements, I understand that the work of health professionals ( ) and education professionals in preventing violence is, first and foremost, a relational process of listening to the other. The coexistence of health professionals with those responsible for the violence creates a space for building a helping relationship that seeks, at every moment, to raise awareness of the importance of a new way of relating to the child, thus establishing healthy living and a break in the cycle of violence.

I think that the global nature of the phenomenon of violence needs to be present in public policy discussions, and that health and education professionals should play the role of facilitators with children; in other words, through socialization and the expression of feelings and problems, there will be a greater chance that parents will see in the attitudes of professionals more appropriate actions in their relationship with children.

The World Report on Violence and Health (2002) focuses on the problem of violence, basing it on the preventive aspects of violence supported by education campaigns, since these interventions stem from the belief that an increase in awareness and understanding of the phenomenon among the general population will result in lower rates of abuse. This occurs either directly, with abusers recognizing their own behavior as abusive and wrong and seeking treatment, or indirectly, through the recognition and reporting of abuse by victims or third parties.

19. REVIEWING THE CATEGORIES

The research carried out based on the testimonies of the aggressor mothers, before and after the educational process, through the workshops, contributed to a more concrete, real, social and human approach to intrafamily violence.

Thus, with a scientific basis, they constitute solid elements for the effective guidance of strategies to prevent the phenomenon.

The analysis of the data, through the subjects' responses, pointed to the need for primary, secondary and tertiary prevention, which implies the need for multi-professional intervention in the field of Education and Health.

The willingness of the aggressors to change their violent behavior towards the children required a stimulus, provided by the work carried out in the workshops, based on reflections on the situations of intrafamily violence experienced in the families.

It can be said that the success of the workshops in achieving their objectives was influenced by the relationship of trust established between the professionals on the team and the family members taking part in the workshops. This was also helped by the fact that the dynamics of the workshops were adapted to the characteristics of the group of mothers studied.

These families adhered to the group's proposal and there were changes in the maternal behaviors mentioned earlier. All the mothers interviewed reported that they no longer resorted to physical punishment; children were referred to nurseries and schools, one participant returned to work and family members who had problems with alcohol and drugs sought specialized care. A pregnant teenager who was part of the workshops, as a member of a family, changed her mind about the birth of the child, because before the workshops she said she wanted to give the baby up for adoption.

From the first meetings, it was possible to see families experiencing different kinds of crises, suffering from drug abuse, unemployment, lack of support from health and education services, among others.

The families were different, but no family type in this study had adequate material living conditions; the different forms of violence against children did not occur randomly, but were associated with the socio-educational profile of the adults responsible for the children. The mothers had low levels of education and information, and this is an influence on the occurrence of intra-family violence, demonstrating the circumstances of great individual, family and social vulnerability common to the families investigated.

Through the interviews, violence was revealed in many forms, from interpersonal to social inequalities, including the multiple problems that these families face in their daily lives, generally adopting the practice of physical punishment with the children as a way of resolving conflicts, as a means of venting the frustrations of everyday life.

In this sense, the nature of the parenting relationship, in terms of symmetry or asymmetry of authority between generations, pedagogical techniques and values in disciplining the child, cannot be disconnected from the nature of the cultural relationship established.

Another common characteristic of the mothers who attended the workshops was the reproduction of the experiences of family violence they had lived through during childhood. In addition to identifying the children as difficult, as problems, they were confused and admitted to being confused about the right way to educate them. After the workshops, they reported a break from these recurring experiences.

Over the course of the meetings, the problem of violence highlighted by the group was analyzed and re-dimensioned. Based on the problematization of the situations presented, they began to live with new possibilities, established a break from violence and created new perspectives for relationships, especially with regard to specific guidelines for the exercise of parenthood.

The work carried out in the workshops made it possible for each participant to understand their share of responsibility for the violent acts, but this individual was accepted by the group, not in the sense of absolving them of responsibility, but of outlining another strategy of action, pointing out other ways of dealing with the relationship.

The workshops, using the methodology of problematization, are intervention programs built in a participatory way, helping to reduce the negative effects that could occur, such as the temporary suspension or definitive loss of power.

The activities developed in these workshops were a concrete and significant result of the fact that the families perceived the child as a person in a peculiar condition in the process of growth and biopsychosocial development, and should be treated, from an educational point of view, with respect, freedom and dignity, without the use of any kind of violence.

The team provided motivation and support to bring about change in the families. Through the various dynamics carried out in the workshops, the healthy aspect was reinforced, as well as reviewing behaviors that needed to change. The work took place in the sense of intense personal and collective valorization, with the recomposition of individual and maternal images, which had been so damaged. The group experience was important for the mothers, as they shared their sufferings, worries, fears, interests, common experiences and alternatives for non-violent behavior.

The workshops addressed issues of care, corporeality and the possibility of self-care in many circumstances throughout life.

I believe that it is right to identify the consequences, investigate the causes and suggest specific solutions, but while it is important to combat the phenomenon itself, it is much more important, effective and safe to combat the causes themselves, and this can only be done effectively through education.

20. FINAL CONSIDERATIONS

At the end of this doctoral thesis, I feel that it has been very important to reflect on the phenomenon of intrafamily violence.

Despite the constant challenges of a long and strenuous journey, it is possible to say that I was able to gain some insight into the repercussions of workshops for educating those responsible for aggression: interfaces between Nursing Education, Health Education and Social Education. It's worth pointing out that the research has by no means exhausted the subject, but that it is a contributory factor in properly tackling the problem. There was an initial concern to better understand the perceptions of those responsible for smacking as a form of education in order to show other ways of approaching the child, but as the work developed, this need grew as it required a position; in other words, there is no way that any researcher can know something, become more aware of the phenomenon and not get involved in order to broaden the focus of action.

Getting to know the phenomenon and recognizing it required, in addition to my position as a researcher, a life choice to take up the cause of combating intrafamily violence, believing in working together to build happier childhoods.

From this experience, it became clear that children were physically punished, verbally pressured, humiliated by their mothers and family members in the name of socialization, for the development of responsibilities, for the acquisition of a good education. Adults use violence to educate children. In this research, we interviewed and focused on individuals who didn't know about other ways of educating, who had little schooling, who didn't have access to other alternatives, who reproduced the environment in which they were brought up, repeating what they had learned in their families of origin, in other words, that beating was a way of educating.

Thus, this dynamic of intra-family violence is associated with social violence. The violent relationship between adult and child in the family cannot be understood without considering the different existential conditions that affect this relationship. I realize that the issue of violence is very complex. The research pointed to the state's abandonment of the family, mainly due to the lack of care policies that effectively responded to the needs of mothers, who felt insecure about the best way to bring up their children. Society demanded standards of conduct, but they didn't know how to act. At the same time as the media publicizes the prohibition of violence, no other educational alternatives are offered.

Through the actions of the team's professionals, the family members obtained a different model of relationship with the child, and we developed strategies for resolving conflicts and imposing limits in a non-violent way, different from the previous model of family functioning.

For the researcher, there is a clear need to involve the community as a whole, so that as many people as possible can get involved in the process of building a society that supports positive values in relation to caring for children and the family. It is important that the people who had the opportunity to take part in the workshops can now act as multipliers in their communities of the Child Protection philosophy.

I believe that one of the important repercussions demonstrated in the work developed through the workshops is the importance of raising group discussion around citizenship and the extension of the social rights of

each and every Brazilian individual, opening up a space favorable to the dissemination of these rights in relation to children, generating a social awareness that favors their widespread protection.

It is necessary, as a proposal for Health Education, to expand this work, removing it from the specificity of the hospital, with a view to greater social insertion.

As a health professional (nurse) and as an educator (university lecturer), I think it's crucial that when I develop my activities, I do so in the most comprehensive way possible, and this has some practical implications. The first of these is the need to awaken ethical, professional and citizenship duties in nursing students, in order to acquire knowledge that contributes to the better quality of professional training, because I believe that the university must be committed to reality, since these students will be faced with this problem on a daily basis in their practice.

In this sense, it is suggested that the results of this study are fundamental for integration into academic curricula in the areas of Education and Health, allowing for a transdisciplinary approach that results in prevention and early intervention programs which, as a priority in this research, were configured as a way of avoiding the risk of recurrences.

The second implication is that this research cannot be considered as a finished task, but as a stimulus that brings up different questions on the subject.

As such, it must be tackled through greater mobilization and integration of different segments of the Hospital's Health Teams, with Teachers, Government Authorities, Representatives of Civil Society Institutions, Social Movements and Communication Professionals, in order to join forces in the face of the Complexity of the phenomenon of violence.

In their evaluations of the workshops, the hospital care team noted the urgent need to involve other professionals who are not yet part of the team, such as a pedagogue and a family therapist.

The workshops made it possible for professionals to understand that violence is an integral part of the very context in which these families live and that, perhaps for this reason, it was so natural and trivialized for them.

The work carried out allowed the participants to be welcomed and respected; the environment was made up of a space for reflection, discussion, acceptance, change and, above all, participation.

It is believed that, with the workshops, both the children's abusers, family members and professionals were able to change some aspects of their lives. There have been changes in attitudes, expressed verbally and concretely, such as improved self-esteem, greater flexibility, greater acceptance of one's own faults and those of others, greater rapport and affection.

In other words, it is necessary to emphasize the importance of the relationships between the various systems, reinforcing the political and educational dimension of the professional in the role of articulator between the various sectors of society, with the aim of involving them in the process in a global way.

Professionals working in the field of social education aim to transform realities. The work carried out in the workshops enabled the group of professionals to understand that family life is a construction of social practice, the product of which is the organization of our own world.

It is easy to see that the prevention of intrafamily violence implies reflecting on what stage each social group is at in relation to the perception of the problem, because the way to intervene is related to the broad political will to formulate specific coping strategies that encompass the various integrated sectors of Health, Education and Justice.

In this sense, I perceive difficulties in approaching the issue of intrafamily violence in terms of the absence of a policy from our state, the deficit of the judicial system to provide adequate, prompt responses to cases of intrafamily violence, the weak commitment between the health and education sectors to identify the problem and generate quick and effective responses. This is probably related to the lack or precariousness of specific training for professionals qualified to work in the area.

Families should find support in institutions, both private and public, so that their members can adequately carry out their duties; in other words, it is essential that all family members can maintain a constant dialogue with health and education professionals, in order to be able to see, in their actions, appropriate references that promote balanced child development.

It is important to recognize the child as a being with full rights, interactive from birth, with basic needs, in which the environment and the child/caregiver bonding process emerge as fundamental elements for harmonious growth, allowing for the development of protective factors in families and thus reducing the number of cases of intra-family violence.

In this sense, the work of the workshops makes it possible to offer support to the family with regard to parenting, especially with specific guidance for mothers, so that they can develop their maternal skills in a desirable way, reducing and/or eradicating the possibilities of occurrence of numerous risks that compromise child growth and development.

I believe that the development of a qualified social support network for the family on a daily basis is a decisive factor and should be made up of specialized technicians (psychologists, social workers, doctors, nurses, teachers, pedagogues) who can regularly monitor each case, proving to be more efficient and effective to the extent of their relational and geographical proximity.

21. REFERENCES

ALGERI, S. Characterization of families of children in situations of violence intrafamiliar. 2001. Dissertation (Master's Degree in Nursing) - Postgraduate Program in Nursing, Federal University of Rio Grande do Sul, 2001.

ALGERI, S.; QUAGLIA, M.; EIDT, O ; Intrafamily violence: proposal for an educational assistance methodology. Development Project. Universidade Federal do Rio Grande do Sul, Hospital de Clinicas de Porto Alegre, Porto Alegre, 2002.

AMEN, D.G. The instruction manual that should come with your child. São Paulo: Mercuryo, 2005.

ANTONI, C. D; KOLLER, S.H. Vulnerability and family resilience: a study with adolescents who have suffered intrafamilial abuse. Revista de Psicologia da PUCRS. Porto Alegre, v.31, n.1, p. 39 -66,jan/jul2000.

APAP, G. et al. The Construction of Knowledge and Citizenship: from the school to the city. Porto Alegre: Artmed, 2002.

ASSIS, S. G. Quando crescer é um desafio social: um estudo socioepidemiologico sobre violência em escolares em Duque de Caxias. Rio de Janeiro: ENSP, 1991.

AZEVEDO, M. A.; GUERRA,V. N. A. Victimized children: the little power syndrome. Sào Paulo: Iglù, 1989.

Childhood and fatal violence in the family. Sào Paulo: Iglù, 1998.

AZEVEDO, M.A; GUERRA , V. N. A. Mania de bater: a punição corporal domèstica de crianças e adolescentes no Brasil. Sào Paulo: Iglù, 2001.

BALESTRERI, R. Citizenship and human rights: a direction for education. Passo Fundo: CAPEC, 1999.

BARDIN, L. Content analysis. 3. ed. Lisbon: Ediçôes 70, 2000.

BARUDY, J. La douleur invisible de l'enfant: approche écosystémique de la maltraitance. Ramonville Saint-Agne: Ères, 1997.

BELLINI , M. Y. B. Archeology of family violence. 2002. Thesis (Doctorate at Serviço Social) - Post-Graduation in Social Work, Pontifical Catholic University of Rio Grande do Sul: Porto Alegre, 2002.

BIEHL, J. I. Children hospitalized for maltreatment: care and the meaning of the experiences of nursing caregivers. 1997. Dissertation (Master's Degree in Nursing) Post-Graduation in Nursing, Federal University of Santa Catarina, 1997.

BLAY, E. Adolescência: uma questão de classe social e gènero. In: LEVISKY, D. L. (org.) Adolescência e violência: consequências da realidade. Sào Paulo: Casa do Psicologo, 2000.

BORDENAVE, J.E.D. What is participation? São Paulo: Editora Brasiliense, 1983.

BORGES, C. Saberes docentes: diferentes tipologias e classificações de um campo de pesquisa. Educaçào & Sociedade, ano XXII, n. 74,59 - 6, Abri/2001.

BRAZIL. Ministry of Health. Child and adolescent statute. ECA. Brasilia: Ministry of Health, 1990.

. National Health Council. Diretrizes e Normas regulamentadoras de pesquisa em seres humanos (Resoluçà 196/96,) Diario oficial da Unià. October 16, 1996: 21082-21085.

BRAZELTON, T. B; SPARROW, J, D. A Criança e a Disciplina : o mètodo Brazelton. Lisbon, Editorial Presença, 2004.

BRAZELTON, T. B; SPARROW, J. D. Discipline: the Brazelton method. Porto Alegre: Artmed, 2005.

BRIGGS, D.C. Your child's self-esteem. São Paulo: Martins Fontes, 2002.

CABRAL, M. A. Prevenção da violência conjugal contra a mulher. Ciência e Saùde Coletiva, Rio de Janeiro, v. 4,n.1, p. 183-91,1999.

CAMARGO, C . L.; BURALLI, K. O. Family violence against children and adolescents. Salvador: Ultragraph, 1998.

CAMINHA, R. M. A Violência e seus danos h criança e ao adolescente. Amparo ao Menor Carente AMENCAR: domestic violence. São Leopoldo: [s.e.J, 1999.

CAMINHA, R. M.A Maltreatment: the scourge of childhood. Cadernos de Extensão Unisinos. São Leopoldo: Unisinos, 2000.

CENTEVILLE, M.; CABRAL, M. A.; ATADIA, S. A. Incidence and most frequent types of punishment applied by parents or guardians to schoolchildren in the city of Campinas, SP. Pediatria Moderna, v. 18, n. 3, p. 99- 105, mar. 1997.

CIRILLO; S.; DI BLASIO, P. Lafamille maltraitante. Paris: ESF, 1989.

COSTA, M., LÓPEZ E. Community health. Barcelona: Martinez Roca, 1986.

COSTA, M., LÓPEZ E. Educacion para la salud: una estrategia para cambiar los estilos de vida. Madrid: Ediciones Piramides, 1996.

CORSI, J. Violencia familiar: una mirada sobre e! grave problema social. Buenos Aires: Paidos, 1995.

CUBERES, M.T.G. Eltallerde lostalleres. Buenos Aires: Estrada, 1989.

DESLANDES, S.F. Atençà às crianças e adolescentes vitimas de violência domèstica: análise de um serviço. Cadernos de Saùde Pùblica, Rio de Janeiro, v. 10, p. 10-5, 1994a.

DESLANDES, S. F. Prevenir a violência: um desafio para profissionais de saùde. Rio de Janeiro: FIOCRUZ/JC, 1994b.

PASTORAL EDITION. Holy Bible. São Paulo: SBCI/Ediçôes Paulinas, 1990.

EIDT, O. R.; BIEHL, J.I e ALGERI, S. Atelier de vivências: um ambiente propicio à construçà do cuidado A criança hospitalizada por maus-tratos. Revista Gaùcha de Enfermagem, Porto Alegre, v. 19, n. 1, p.47-55, jan. 1998.

ENGELS, F. El origen de la familia, la propriad y el estado. 9. ed. Buenos Aires: Claridad, 1971.

ELSEN, I. Welcome Speech. Revista Texto e Contexto, familia e violência. Florianopolis, v. 8, number 2, p. 25-28, May to August 1999.

ELSEN, I. Violence knocks on the door. In: LUZ, A. M.H; MANCIA, J.R; MOTTA, M. da G.C. As Amarras da Violência a família, as instituições e a Enfermagem. Brasilia: Brazilian Nursing Association, 2004.

FARINATTI, F.; BIAZUS, D. B.; LEITE, M. B. THE victimized child. Revista Mèdica Santa Casa, ano IV, n. 7, p. 684-89, 1992.

. Social pediatrics and abused children. Rio de Janeiro: MEDSI, 1993.

FERRARI, D. C. A. Diàlogo. Journal of Religious Education. Sào Paulo, ano 11, n.5, p.13-20, mar. 1997.

FLORES, R.Z., MATTOS, L.F.C., SALZANO, F.M. Incest: frequency, predisposing factors, and effects in a brazilian population. Curret Anthropology, 39:554-558, 1998.

FREIRE, P. Pedagogia da esperança: um reencontro com a pedagogia do oprimido. 3. Ed Sào Paulo: Paz e Terra, 1994.

FURNISS, T. Child Sexual Abuse. A multidisciplinary approach. Porto Alegre: Artes Médicas, 1993.

GAUER, R. M.C.; GAUER, G. I. A Fenomenologia da violência. Curitiba: Juruà, 1999.

GADOTTI, M.; GUTIERREZ, F. Community education and popular economy. Sào Paulo: Cortez, 1993. v25.

GOLDANI, A. M. As familias brasileiras: mudanças e perspectivas. Cadernos de Pesquisa, Sào Paulo, n. 91, p, 5-6, nov, 1994.

GOLDIM, J. R. Manual de iniciaçà à pesquisa em saù. 2. 4. rev. ampl. Porto Alegre: Dacasa, 2000,

GOMES, C. G. FILHO, W. D. L. Banalization of Violence in the Family. In: LUZ,AM.H;

MANCIA, J.R; MOTTA, M. da G.C. As Amarras da Violência a familia, as instituições e a Enfermagem. Brasilia: Brazilian Nursing Association, 2004.

GONZALEZ, M. I. S. Health Education for the 21st Century: Communication and Health. Madrid: Diaz de Santos, 1998.

GREEN, AH. Child sexual abuse and incest. In: LEWIS, M. (org.) Tratado de Psiquiatria da infància e da Adolescência. Porto Alegre: Artes Médicas, p.1032-1042, 1995.

GUERRA, V. N. A. Violence between parents and children. Sào Paulo: Cortez, 1985.

Parental violence against children: the tragedy revisited. São Paulo: Cortez, 1998.

HAWLEY, D. DEHAAN, L. Toward a definition of family resilience: integrating life span and family perspectives. Family Process, 35, 283-398, 1996.

HAGUETTE, T. Metodologias Qualitativas na Sociologia. Petrópolis/Rio de Janeiro:

Vozes, 1987.

HELLER, A Instinct, aggression and character. Barcelona: Ediciones Peninsula, 1994.

HOSPITAL DE CLiNICAS DE PORTO ALEGRE. Annual Report 1999. Porto Alegre, 2000. 66 p.

JAEGER, F. P. Education and violence in oppressed families. 2003. Dissertation (Master's Degree in Social and Personality Psychology) - Postgraduate Program in Psychology, Pontifical Catholic University of Rio Grande do Sul, Porto Alegre, 2003.

KAPLAN, H.; SADOCK, R; GREBB, J. Compendium of dynamic psychiatry. 3. ed. PortoAlegre: Artes Médicas, 1997.

LIBÂNEO, J. C. Didatica. Sào Paulo: Cortez, 1994.

LOPEZ, M. R. Fundamentos de la educación social. Madrid: Editorial Sintesis, 2000.

LÜDKE, M. ; ANDRÉ, M. E. D. Pesquisa em Educaçào: abordagens qualitativas. Sào Paulo: EPU, 1986.

MALDONADO, M. T. Os construtores da paz: caminhos da preservaçao da violência. São Paulo: Moderna, 1997.

MACALIIAES, T. Maltreatment of children and young people. Practical guide for professionals. Coimbra: Quarteto, 2004.

MARTINS, M. R. S. Maltreatment and Sexual Abuse: the family universe. Bertholdo Weber Center for the Defense of Children and Adolescents. São Leopoldo, 1997, p.29-32.

MENEGHEL, S. N. Violence in childhood and adolescence. Jornal de Pediatria, v. 71, n. 6, p. 294-96, 1995.

. Families in pieces: a study on domestic violence and aggression in adolescence. 1996. Thesis (Doctorate in Medicine) - Graduate School of Medicine, Federal University of Rio Grande do Sul, Porto Alegre, 1996.

MENEGHEL, S. N; et al. Violent daily life: mental health promotion workshops. Ciência e Saùde Coletiva, Rio de Janeiro, v.5, n.1, p.1-16, 2000.

MINAYO, M. C. S. Bibliografia comentada da produção cientifica brasileira sobre violência e saù. Rio de Janeiro: National School of Public Health, 1990.

. Social research in health. Sào Paulo: Cortez, 1992.

. Social violence from a public health perspective. Caderno Saùde Pùblica, Rio de Janeiro, v. 10, n. supl, p. 7-18, 1994.

MINAYO, M. C. S.; ASSIS, S. Violence and health in childhood and adolescence: an agenda for strategic research. Saùde em Debate. n.39, p.58-63, 1993.

MINAYO, M. C. S.; SOUZA, E. R. Violência sob o Olhar da Saùde: a infrapolitica da contemporaneidade brasileira. Rio de Janeiro: Fiocruz, 2003.

MINISTRY OF HEALTH. Multiplier manual: adolescents. Secretariat for Special Health Projects. National Coordination of Sexually Transmitted Diseases - AIDS. Brasilia, 1997.

MINISTRY OF HEALTH. Intrafamilial violence: guidelines for in-service practice. Secretariat of Health Policies. Cadernos de AtençBo Basica n. 8. Brasilia, 2001.

HEALTH MINISTRY. Notification of maltreatment of children and adolescents by health professionals, one step closer to citizenship in health. Secretariat of Health Care. Normas e Manuais Técnicos n. 167. Brasilia, 2002.

MORAIS, E. P, Enfermagem e familia: evitar a negligência. Santa Maria: [s.e], 1999.

MORAIS, E. P. ; EIDT, O.R. Knowing to avoid: negligence in health care for children and adolescents. Revista Gaùcha de Enfermagem. Porto Alegre, v.20, n. esp., p.6-2 1, 1999.

MORAIS, R. Violence and education. Campinas: Papirus, 1995.

MOSQUERA, J.J.M. ; STOBAUS, C. D.; Education for Health: a challenge for changing societies. 2ed. Porto Alegre: Luzzatto, 1984.

MUSZKAT, M. Intrafamily violence: new forms of intervention. In: LEVISKY, D.L. (org). Adolescence and violence: community actions in prevention. Sâo Paulo: Casa do PsicologoZHebraica, 2002,

MUZA, G. M. The abused and neglected child. Jornal de Pediatria, v. 70, n. 1, p. 56-60, 1994.

NEDER, G. Violência e Cidadania. Porto Alegre: Sèrio Antonio Fabris Editor, 1994.

NEWELL, P. Children are people too. The case against physical punishment. London: Bedford Square Press, 1989.

NITSCHKE, R. G. A journey through the imaginary world of being a healthy family in everyday life in post-modern times: the discovery of bonds of affection as a path. 1999. Thesis (Doctorate in Nursing) - Post-Graduation in Nursing, Federal University of Santa Catarina: Florianopolis, 1999.

OLIVEIRA, W. F. Educaçào social de rua: as bases politicas e pedagogicas para uma educaçà popular. Porto Alegre: Artes Médicas, 2004.

OMER, H. Autoridade sem Violência: o resgate da voz dos pais. Belo Horizonte: Arte Sà, 2002.

OSKI, F. A. Principios e Pràtica de Pediatria. Rio de Janeiro: Guanabara Koogan, 1992.

OSORIO, L. C. Familia hoje. Porto Alegre: Artes Médicas, 1996.

PEDRO, E. N.R. Experiences and (con)experiences of children with HIV/AIDS and their families: educational implications.2000. Thesis (Doctorate in Education) - Post-Graduation in Education, Pontifical Catholic University of Rio Grande do Sul: Porto Alegre, 2000.

POLIT, D.F.; HUNGLER, B. P. Fundamentals of Nursing Research. Porto Alegre: Artes Médicas, 1995.

PRADO, L. P. et al. Lithium reduces abusive maternal behavior: a preliminary report. Journal of Clinical Pharmacy and Therapeutics 11-26,p. 1-4, 2001.

QUAGLIA, M. C.; MARQUES, M,F. Course: social work intervention in situations of domestic violence against children and adolescents. Porto Alegre: HCPA/UFRGS, 2000 (mimeo).

RBS LAUNCHES CHILD PROTECTION CAMPAIGN. Zero Hora, year 40, n. 13.805, p. 4-10,8 jun. 2003.

WORLD REPORT on Violence and Health. KRUG EG et al., eds. Geneva, World Health Organization, 2002.

REPORT for the End of Punishments against Children: the European experience.

Report of the Legislative Assembly. Porto Alegre: Citizenship and Human Rights Commission of Rio Grande do Sul, 1996. 103p.

ROSARIO, M.D. Politicas Pùblicas voltadas para a Proteç5o de Crianças e Adolescentes Vitimas de Violência. Support for Children in Need of Domestic Violence. São Leopoldo, p.12-17, 1999.

SANTOS, C. S. Violência em tempo de globalização. São Paulo: HUCITEC, 1999.

SANTOS, B. C.; et al. Mistreatment and sexual abuse of children and adolescents: a profile of the situation in the state of Rio Grande do Sul. São Leopoldo: CEDECA, Bertholdo Weber, 1998.

SANTOS, J. V. T. A cidadania dilacerada. Zero Hora newspaper, Porto Alegre, p. 4, August 24, 1996, Life section.

. Violence: citizenship torn apart. In: REPORT OF THE MUNICIPAL CONFERENCE ON HUMAN RIGHTS, Porto Alegre, p. 2735, May 1998.

SANTOS, C. S.; ALGERI, S. The abused child: from prevention to rehabilitation. In CONGRESSO BRASILEIRO DE ENFERMAGEM, 46. Porto Alegre, 1994 (mimeo).

STAKE,R. E. Investigacion con estudio de caso. Madrid: Morata, 1998.

TIBA, I. Sejafeliz meu filho. São Paulo: Editora Gente, 1995.

TIBA, I. Who loves, educates! São Paulo: Editora Gente, 2002.

THOMPSON, E. D.; ASHWILL, J.W. An Introduction to Pediatric Nursing. Porto Alegre: Artes Médicas, 1996.

UNESCO. Education: a treasure to be discovered. Report for UNESCO of the International Commission on Education for the 21st Century. Sâo Paulo: Cortez, 2000.

VARELA, Z.M. de V. The family in real or potential situations of domestic violence. In: LUZ, A. M.H; MANCIA, J.R; MOTTA, M.da G.C. As Amarras da Violência a familia, as instituições e a Enfermagem. Brasilia: Brazilian Nursing Association, 2004.

VIEIRA, E.; VOLQUND, L. Teaching Workshops: What? Why? How? Porto Alegre: EDIPUCRS, 2002.

VISSING, Y.M. Verbal aggression by parents and psychosocial problems y children. Child abuse and neglect. NewYork: Seribner, 1991.

WAIDMAN, M. A. P.; DECESARO, M. das N.; MARCOS, S.S. Living with family violence. In: LUZ, A. M.H; MANCIA, J.R; MOTTA, M. da G.C. As Amarras da Violência a familia, as instituições e a Enfermagem. Brasilia: Brazilian Nursing Association, 2004,

WEfALEY, L. F.; WONG, D. L. Pediatric Nursing. Essential Elements for Effective Intervention. Rio de Janeiro: Guanabara Koogan, 1989.

ZAGURY, T. Educating without guilt. The genesis of ethics. Rio de Janeiro: Record, 2002.

ZAGURY, T. Limits without Trauma. Building Citizens. Rio de Janeiro: Record, 2001.

ZANELA, L. After all, whose ball is it? Zero Hora, year 40, n. 13.805, p.13, October 4, 2004.

22. LEARN

APPENDIX A - IDENTIFICATION FORM

DIMENSION: SOCIODEMOGRAPHIC	
1. Percapita Family Income	In minimum wages: 1()1s 2()2s 3 ( )3s/+
2. Place of residence	1 ( ) Porto Alegre 2 ( ) Metropolitan Region 3 ( ) Inland Rio Grande do Sul 4 ( ) Other
3. Housing conditions (basic sanitation)	1()Yes 2()No 3()$^{⅞(ua)}$ 4 ( ) Drainage
Type of dwelling (construction material, number of parts)	1 ( ) Masonry 2 ( ) Wood 3 ( ) Other Which one: ___ ( ) Pieces: Number _________
5. Getting Mothers into the Labor Market	1 ( ) Never worked 2 ( ) Employed in the formal market 3 ( ) Participant in the informal market 4 ( ) Unemployed 5 ( ) Retired
6. Father's integration into the job market	1 ( ) Never worked 2 ( ) Employed in the formal market 3 ( ) Participant in the informal market 4 ( ) Unemployed 5 ( ) Retired
7. Mother's schooling	1 ( ) Illiterate Elementary School 2 ( ) incomplete 3 ( ) complete Secondary Education 4 ( ) incomplete 5 ( ) complete Higher education 6 ( ) incomplete 7 ( ) complete
8 Father's schooling	1 ( ) Illiterate Elementary School 2 ( ) incomplete 3 ( ) complete Secondary Education 4 ( ) incomplete 5 ( ) complete Higher education 6 ( ) incomplete 7 ( ) complete
9. Age of the aggressor	9 ( ) Years

10. Parents' age	()Dad ( ) Mother
11. Number of family members	()П)²()³()(4)()(5)()(+5) ______ .... ______
12. Relationship to Abuser (a)	1()Father 2() Stepfather 3 ( ) Mother 4 ( ) Stepmother 5 ( ) Family member. Who? ______ 6 ( ) Neighbor or Friend 7 ( )Unknown
13. Family illness	1 ( ) Absent 2 ( ) Present Type of illness: ( ) Physics ()Aguda ( ) Chronic ( ) Mental ()Aguda ( ) Conical
14. Family pattern of drug use	1 ( ) Absent 2 ( ) Present, specify Alcohol Loló Marijuana Cocaine Crack Other. Which ones?

APPENDIX B - PRE-WORKSHOP INTERVIEW

Perceptions of children's guardians about spanking as a way of
of educating

Interview guide

1. What ways of educating children do you know? What do you think about them?
2. In your opinion, what does the child do to be punished?
3. When the child has that behavior you told me before, how do you act? Do you think it works?
4. How did your parents punish you when you were a child?

APPENDIX C - OBSERVATION FORM

Elements to be Considered for the Observed Behaviors, contained in the workshop observation report :

a. verbal
b. non-verbal (mimicry, posture)

c. behavioral

d. level of activity/participation

APPENDIX D - POST-WORKSHOP INTERVIEW

1. How was your participation in the workshop?
2. Do you remember the subjects covered in the workshops? Please comment.
3. Was it important for you to take part in the workshops? Why was it important?
4. Do you think that taking part in the workshops has helped your relationship with your child? Please explain.
5. And at home, with other family members?

APPENDIX E - SYMBOL CONSTELLATION WORKSHOP

The first meeting of the workshop was the day to introduce the group members who would be taking part, i.e. the perpetrators' guardians and the multi-professional team that would be taking part and coordinating the work of the workshops.

The initial idea was for people to introduce themselves and realize the importance of being part of that group, made up of people in a working group to reflect on, discuss and intervene in intrafamily violence.

The team was clear that one of the fundamental goals of the work would be to make families aware of the violence they were using against their children so that, during the meetings, they could propose actions to change this behavior.

The dynamic used in the first meeting was called The Constellation of Symbols. All the participants, family members and staff were sitting in chairs arranged in a circle. The nurse began the dynamic by introducing herself to the group and explaining that she would be coordinating the meeting that day.

The group was asked if anyone knew what was in the suitcase in the nurse's hands. The group was encouraged to come up with ideas. The proposal was explained. All the participants, one at a time, had to go to the center of the circle and pick up the object that most identified with their personality and, through it, introduce themselves to the group.

After the opinions had been collected, one of the mothers, assisted by the nurse, opened the case which was placed on a table in the center of the circle.

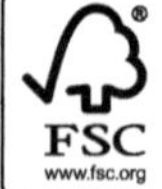

MIX
Papier aus verantwortungsvollen Quellen
Paper from responsible sources
FSC® C105338

Printed by Books on Demand GmbH, Norderstedt / Germany